Eat It All
by
Eating Right

The Stavros Method
An Alternative to Dieting

by Stavros Mastrogiannis

Eat It All by Eating Right
The Stavros Method
An Alternative to Dieting

by Stavros Mastrogiannis

Live Your Way Thin Publications

Dedication

This book is dedicated to the fight against obesity and to the millions of people who are trying to balance life, weight loss, and staying healthy. The purpose of this book is to provide these people with the ammunition they need to finally win their weight loss battle.

Disclaimer

The author recommends talking to your doctor and getting a full physical before starting any exercise and/or diet program. The medical community has varying opinions on proper nutrition, improving health, and losing weight. This book contains the opinions of the author, and is for reference and informational purposes only. It is in no way intended as medical counseling or medical advice. The activities, physical or otherwise, described herein are for informational purposes only, and may be too strenuous or dangerous for some people. Please consult with your doctor before engaging in them. The author and the publisher cannot be held liable for any injury caused, or alleged to be caused, directly or indirectly, by the information contained in this book.

Table of Contents

Stavros Mastrogiannis

Foreword

Oh no, not another diet book!

I wouldn't blame anyone if that was their initial reaction when they first heard about this new book. There are thousands and thousands of diet books on the market today, and yet we are losing the weight loss battle. So, how can one more diet book make any difference?

It's very simple. This is not a diet book; it's an alternative to dieting. You see, most diet books give you a list of foods you should eat, a list of foods you should not eat, how many calories you should consume and how often (according to the clock) you should eat. They also expect you that you will be able to incorporate all their suggestions into your life at once, assuming that once you see results, you will be motivated to stick to the diet. Well, this book is nothing like that. As you might already be aware of, that approach has not worked so far and it never will, and here is why. When a diet eliminates an entire food group, it actually increases your desire for that food. It's in human nature to want what we can't have, so if a diet tells you to eliminate a certain food, it just places more emphasis on that food. In my approach no food is off limits.

In addition, diets like to label foods as healthy or unhealthy, fattening or non-fattening. The fact is, how food affects our health and weight is not determined only by the nutritional value of the food. How fast and how well you chewed your food, how much you ate, and whether you were genuinely hungry when you started eating, also have a great influence on how food affects us.

Let me prove it to you. Back in October 2011, I did a very interesting experiment. For two months, Monday through Friday, I ate all my meals at fast food restaurants, mostly McDonalds. The foods I was eating were definitely considered unhealthy and fattening, and yet by the end of the two months I lost 3 lbs (I was not looking to lose weight), my cholesterol went down (although it was already very good), and my triglycerides also went down (again, they were very good to begin with). How can that be? Didn't Morgan Spurlock, in his documentary *Super Size Me*, show that eating at McDonalds is bad for your health and weight? The difference is, that unlike Mr. Spurlock who ate breakfast, lunch, and dinner regardless of whether he was hungry, and who ate all of the food they gave him for each meal regardless of whether he would have been satisfied with less, I listened to my body.

During my experiment I followed 3 simple rules. I ate only when I was hungry, I ate slowly and mindfully, and I stopped eating when I had satisfied my hunger. So you see, although Mr. Spurlock and I were eating similar foods, we got completely different results. You can go to the most health-conscious restaurant and eat the way Mr. Spurlock ate in *Super Size Me*, and I bet you would get similar unhealthy results. I don't want anybody to misunderstand me, I am not for or against fast food restaurants, all I'm trying to say is that *how* we eat can affect our health and weight as much as *what* we eat. There are more details about this experiment later in this book.

Another thing you will learn from my program (The Stavros Method) that you will not learn from any other diet book, is how to eat the right amount of food without counting calories. Counting calories is a very unrealistic way to lose weight. Yes, we can keep track of the number of calories we eat, but sooner or later we get tired of doing it and stop. The good news is, there is an alternative to counting calories, and that is learning to listen to your body. Your body can tell you when you need to eat and when you've had enough food. The trick is to learn to pay attention to your body's signals, and that is exactly what you will learn from this program. Another major difference between my approach to better eating habits and all other diet books is that I won't try to change all your eating habits at once. Although changing all your eating habits at once will produce fast results, it also almost always leads to burnout and, eventually, regaining all the weight. Think about it: most diets have you make all necessary dietary changes all at once. How is that working for most people? Let me tell you, not very well. According to The National Institutes of Health, 98% of people who lose weight gain it back. Actually, I don't think I needed to quote any studies; all you have to do is look around you. How many people do you know who lost weight and gained it back? Perhaps it even happened to you. It is almost impossible to make so many changes to your eating habits all at once and not get overwhelmed, no matter how good your initial results are. Unless you have super-strong willpower, sooner or later you will return to your old habits and regain the weight. The best way, and for most people the only way to lose weight and keep it off, is to lose weight by making small sustainable changes in our dietary habits over time, and that is the way this book will help you lose the weight you need to lose.

I have found that most people need to make 3 to 7 changes in their eating habits in order to lose weight and improve their health. Instead of taking the approach that most other diet books have taken, which is basically to apply all the dietary changes at once, I have broken down everything you must do into 7 Simple Steps. All you have to do is focus on completing each step before moving to the next one. By the time you go through all 7 Simple Steps, you will have developed all the necessary eating habits you need to lose the weight you want and — more importantly — improve your health in the process.

The bottom line is, whatever dietary changes you make in order to lose weight have to become habitual (require little or no conscious thought), if you want to keep the weight off. If you constantly have to fight temptations and constantly have to be thinking about what you can eat, what you can't eat, and how many calories you need, sooner or later you will burn out and revert to your old habits.

Take the first step today toward a leaner and healthier body by reading this book. You will be surprised how easy it is to change your eating habits if you do it the right way and you have the right attitude.

My suggestion is to first read the whole book from cover to cover, to get an understanding of my overall philosophy on nutrition. It is important that you understand the benefits of everything I will be asking you to do throughout the program, because if you don't fully understand why you should be take a certain action, you will not be as motivated to take that action, and sooner or later you will talk yourself out of taking the action, and quit. So please read the entire book, to get a clear understanding of my overall philosophy before taking the steps for change. You will be so much more motivated once you understand the importance of what you are doing.

Once you are ready to begin, make sure you have completed all the prerequisites before taking the first step of changing your body and health forever. They will make a huge difference. All the prerequisites are explained in Section 12.

Stavros Mastrogiannis

Section 1: Weight Gain is a Blessing

You're probably thinking I have lost my mind, but once I explain why weight gain is a blessing, I'm sure you will agree with me. Many people believe that because they are thin, they don't have to worry about their diet — that only people who have a weight problem need to think about what they eat. These thin people should think again. Being thin does not mean junk food has no ill effects on you. All it means is that your body can burn, or not observe, the extra calories, so your weight does not increase. However, you still can develop heart disease, diabetes, or any other disease that overweight people develop.

The reason I consider weight gain a blessing is the fact that, at the very least, people who gain weight when they eat poorly and/or don't exercise get a clear message in the mirror that tells them, *you are doing something wrong*, whereas a thin person often does not get that message until it's too late.

Due to the fact that thin people don't see any dramatic physical consequences in the mirror due to their bad eating habits or lack of exercise, often a thin person will find it much harder to improve his or her diet and start an exercise program than someone who gains weight easily. A thin person doesn't have that extra motivation to look good in a bathing suit because he or she looks fine now, and can't see what bad habits are doing to their health on the inside.

So you see, if you are overweight and you gain weight easily, you should consider yourself lucky to have an obvious warning that's telling you to take action *now*.

Section 2:
Why We Can't Keep Weight Off
After We Lose It

These days we can't turn on the TV or look at a magazine without seeing an ad for some weight loss product or service. One would think, with all those weight loss products and services on the market today, we would be the thinnest nation in the world, but we're not! Americans spend billions of dollars per year on weight loss products and services, and yet we are still losing the weight loss battle. There are many reasons why we have not been able to lose weight, or to be more precise, to lose weight and keep it off. Here I will talk about what I consider the number one reason for this.

I would like to start with a question. What is the one thing most weight loss products and services on the market today have in common? They promise fast results. The reason they promise fast results is because that's what people want to hear. They don't take into consideration the fact that fast results are almost impossible to maintain for the long term, but then again, the ads only promise that we will lose the weight fast, not that we'll be able to keep it off. Most weight loss products can deliver on their promise of fast results, but where they fail miserably is in delivering permanent results.

Let me explain the reason why they fail at helping people lose weight permanently. Here is an undisputed fact: In order to lose weight fast, you must make big changes in your life. There is no way around this fact. The problem with big changes is that they take us far outside our comfort zone. The farther away you get from your comfort zone, the more likely you will get overwhelmed and quit.

Humans are creatures of habit. The majority of the things we do every day require little or no active thought on our part. When we do the things we have always done, things we know we can do, we are inside our comfort zone. If we want to change our habits, or add a new habit, we need to take ourselves out of "automatic gear" and consciously practice the new habit, which requires more energy on our part. Whether that energy is mental or physical does not matter, because either way, when we're trying to implement a new habit in our everyday lives, that new action takes us outside our comfort zone, which makes us feel uncomfortable, and our bodies fight to get us back into the comfort zone. Of course, by repeating the new action, eventually the comfort zone expands to include that new action.

The question is, can you keep repeating the new action and tolerate the discomfort long enough for that new action to become a habit and become incorporated in your comfort zone? Also keep in mind that the more new habits we're trying to develop at once, the bigger the discomfort we will feel and the longer it will take for our comfort zone to expand to include the new habits, which means we have a greater chance of burning out. It's important to implement change one small step at a time.

Unfortunately, most weight loss programs and diets on the market today simply don't understand how habits are formed and how people's comfort zones work — or they just don't care, because all they want is to make a quick buck. They wrongly assume that once we start seeing results we'll be motivated to stick with their diet or weight loss program. Wrong! If results were enough to motivate us, then why can't most people keep the weight off after they lose it? Statistics show that the vast majority of people regain lost weight within two to five years.

The main reason we regain the weight is because most weight loss programs and diets ask us to make many big changes all at once. They fail to understand how to introduce and apply change into our lives without overwhelming us. This book will not only tell you what actions to take for better health and permanent weight loss, it will also teach you how to develop those actions into everyday habits.

Section 3: How to Lose Weight and Keep it Off

The best way to lose weight is through small, sustainable changes over time. If you want to keep the weight off, the actions required to lose the weight have to become automatic *habits* and part of your comfort zone. Actually, the process of losing weight permanently is much easier than losing weight quickly, because you only need to make small changes at any one time. Each week your focus should be on the habit or habits you are trying to develop, not the weight you are trying to lose. In Section 12, you'll learn how to incorporate all the healthy eating habits you will learn in this book, in a way that will not overwhelm you. As you're working through the steps, it's important to remember that your excess weight is only a symptom of a problem. The true problem is the habits that made you overweight in the first place.

By following the 7 Simple Steps in Section 12, you'll lose weight more slowly, but you will only need to lose the weight once, whereas with most of the weight loss programs and diets on the market today, you'd end up having to lose the same weight over and over again every year. What's the point of losing weight fast, if you're going to gain it all back again? Wouldn't you rather take a few extra months, lose the weight the right way, and never worry about your weight again for the rest of your life?

Section 4: Let's Make Junk Food Special Again

First of all, let's talk about what I mean by "junk food." My definition of junk food is any food that is highly processed, high in refined carbs (white flour and/or sugar), has little or no nutritional value, and that is eaten for the sheer pleasure of it. Examples of junk foods include, but are not limited to, white bread, cake, ice cream, doughnuts, cookies, milkshakes, high-sugar salad dressings and dips, soda, candy, desserts, chips of any kind, most alcoholic drinks (more than one per sitting), etc. By the way, merely adding vitamins to a food does not take it off the list of junk foods. Notice, pizza and burgers did not make the list. Just because a food is high in fat does not make it a junk food. In Greece we used to eat the skin of the pig which was 100% fat and we did not have a weight problem. Once you learn *how to eat*, you will see that fat will not have any effect on your weight or health.

One of the things most diets have in common is that they want you to eat certain foods and completely eliminate others, usually junk foods. However, these diets don't take into account the human psychology behind wanting something you can't have. Have you ever watched a child play with one toy while completely ignoring another toy lying nearby? As soon as another child picks up that toy, all of a sudden the first child wants it. It's human nature to want what we can't have, therefore trying to eliminate certain foods only draws attention to the foods we can no longer have. And let's face it; most "bad" foods taste good.

Most diets tell you to eliminate all junk food from your diet so you can lose weight fast. Most people do exactly that, and lose weight. However, since we often want what we can't have, it's only a matter of time before we give in to an inevitable craving.

When we do, we say to ourselves, "I cheated already. I feel guilty anyway, so I might as well have all the junk food I want today. Tomorrow I'll be extra good to make up for today."
That is how binge eating starts. The fear of not being able to have a certain food can cause us to binge on that food. Before we know it, we start breaking the diet more often, especially when the number on the scale starts moving up. We eventually give up, and by that time, we may even have established a habit of binge eating.

So you see, by simply saying "no" to junk food, all we do is make ourselves want it even more. If it were that easy to give up junk food, the junk food companies would be out of business by now! In Greece we had our fair share of junk food with no major consequences to our health. Why? Because junk food was special. We did not have it all the time, and when we did, most of the time we were hungry. As you will learn later in this book, when you eat only when you are hungry, at least most of the time, you body is better able to deal with not-so-healthy food. So, my rule is to make junk food special and have it only on the weekends and special occasions. This way and you will get to enjoy your favorite junk food guilt-free and you get to enjoy a healthier and leaner body. Even the unhealthiest food on the planet will not affect you the same way if you eat it when you are truly hungry. We will learn more about this in a later section of this book.

In the next section, I will explain in detail how to take control of yourself and develop the habit of eating junk food only on the weekends and special occasions.

Section 5: Control Yourself, Not Your Environment

Another big mistake we make when trying to lose weight is cleaning out our cupboards. We eliminate all the foods we're not supposed to eat by getting them out of the house. I even hear nutritionists recommending this approach, with the idea that their clients will not be tempted to cheat. This sounds like good advice on the surface, but it does not teach us one very important thing: self-control.

I lived in Greece for 12 years before moving to the U.S., where, over a long period and before I knew any better, I picked up many bad eating habits. I never had a weight problem, but when I got into the fitness field I realized that not gaining weight didn't necessarily mean that junk food had no ill effect on my body. That's when I tried to change the bad eating habits I had picked up over the years.

On my first attempt, I did what most people do. I eliminated from my house all my favorite junk foods and sodas and told myself I would never have them again. The problem I found with this method was, every time I encountered my favorite junk foods somewhere else, say, at a party, I would binge on them. After eating only one piece of food that was on the "forbidden" list, I'd tell myself, "Oh well, I broke my rule. Might as well enjoy all the junk food I can have now, and tomorrow I will be extra good with my diet to make up for today."

This would happen two or three times each week because, as you know, junk food is everywhere. In this way, I learned that trying to control my environment (in this case, by removing all the junk food from my house) does not work.

I started looking at people who were successful, not just in weight loss, but in business and in life, and what I found out was this: People who are successful in their endeavors don't eliminate all temptation from their lives. What they do is learn to make themselves to do the right thing, in spite of all the temptations around them.

Weight loss is no different. You must learn to control yourself, not your environment, because the fact is, you can't always control your environment. You can eliminate all the tempting foods from your house, but can you do the same for your work environment? Most people that I've talked to say this is not possible, since co-workers frequently bring candy and other sweets to share at work.

So my question then became, how can I learn to control myself? It took a little time, but after a few more failed attempts, I came up with a method by which I was able to take complete control of my eating habits, and had absolutely no problem resisting food temptations of all kinds. I could go to a party where they had all my favorite sweets, have a great time, and not have even one sweet. Most importantly, I did not feel deprived. I kept all my favorite cookies in my house without feeling the urge to eat one. Here's how I did it.

It started with the realization that having *some* junk food will not kill us. After all, we ate junk food in Greece when I lived there and we were very healthy and thin. My school in Greece had about 350 kids and, out of all those kids, only three or four were overweight. I thought cancer was a rare disease because I didn't know anyone — or even know anyone who *knew* anyone — who had cancer. The average 80-year-old person was completely independent and fully functioning; I had never seen a walker and not even many canes. People lived long and healthy lives, and yet still ate some junk food.

But here is the difference: We did not eat it every day. We

usually reserved it for special occasions. For instance, about once each week, when there was a good movie on TV, my mother gave us potato chips and Coke as a snack to eat during the movie. Although there was always soda at our celebrations and holiday parties, there was no soda during our regular lunch or dinners. There was no dessert after dinner — only when we went to a restaurant did we have dessert. At home, dessert was usually apples or oranges. Only on holidays did my mother make those delicious Greek desserts, like baklava and galaktoboureko.

Nowadays if you go to Greece, people have become very overweight, including the kids. What changed? Among other things, junk food has gone from being a treat eaten once in a while to something indulged in every day, and most of the time on top of a regular meal.

The point I'm trying to make is that we don't need to eliminate all the junk food from our lives to be thin and healthy. All we need to do is treat junk foods as they were meant to be treated — as a treat. In other words, we need to make junk food special, like it used to be. Once I realized that, I was able to come up with a plan to help myself put junk food in its proper place in our diet, as a treat. Here's how I made junk food special again.

I started with soda. I was a very heavy soda drinker, and knew that if I simply tried to eliminate soda from my diet, it wouldn't work — cravings would sabotage my effort. Instead, I made a rule that I could not have any soda Monday through Friday, but I could have all the soda I wanted on weekends, starting at 5 p.m. on Friday. This made my weekend more special. I told my family — and I have a big family — that I would be required to give $20 to anyone who saw me drinking soda, including diet soda, during the week before 5 p.m. on Friday.

The first week was hard, but because I could have all the soda I wanted on the weekend, I found it much easier to resist temptation during the week. Whenever I had a craving for soda, I said to myself, "I should wait to have soda this weekend so I can enjoy it, without feeling guilty about it afterwards."

That first weekend, I drank plenty of soda to make up for not having it all week. I must say, I enjoyed my soda much more because I did not feel guilty about drinking it. On Monday, again I stopped drinking soda until 5 p.m. on Friday. This time it was much easier to resist drinking soda.

Whenever I felt a craving, I dismissed it as soon as it came up. I said to myself, "It's a weekday, and on weekdays I don't drink soda." I didn't dwell on the fact that I could not have the soda I craved. I just moved on, and thought about something else, or engaged in an activity that left no room for thoughts about the food I craved. I found that by dismissing the craving right away, the craving lost its power over me.

That weekend I drank soda again, but not as much as I'd had the previous week. Once I became comfortable with the knowledge of being able to have all the soda I wanted every weekend, I did not have the urge to drink soda during the week. When Monday came around, not having soda was not as big of a deal. My thinking started to change. I didn't have as many cravings during the week, but when I did, I only needed to remind myself, "This is a weekday; I don't have soda on weekdays." Because I did not give myself a choice and didn't dwell on the fact that I couldn't have soda, the cravings lost their power over my thoughts.

When the third weekend came and went, on Monday I realized I hadn't had any soda on the weekend — I didn't even miss it. I gave myself few more weeks to fully adopt the rule of no soda Monday through 5 p.m. Friday before I started working on the next rule.

The next rule I worked on was to avoid any type of sweets or candy from Monday morning through 5 p.m. Friday. I set a clear definition of what I considered "sweets and candy," and got to work.

It has been over seven years since I established these eating habits, and I now have a few sodas per month and some form of candy or sweets most weekends. The rule of "no sodas or candy during the week" is so ingrained in me that I hardly ever get any cravings during the week. My habit of not eating sweets on weekdays is so ingrained that if I'm at a birthday party during the week, I don't even feel the need to have cake (unless, of course, it's my own birthday). Ever since I made junk foods special, indulging in them on the weekends or special occasions only, I enjoy them much more. The best thing is, I don't feel guilty after I have them.

More importantly, I feel great during the week, which is when I have to be at my best. And, because I allow myself to indulge in some junk food every weekend, I don't feel deprived. Remember, your body can tolerate a certain amount of not-so-good food. As long as you eat healthfully and for the right reasons the rest of the time and, of course, exercise regularly, you'll be able to maintain great health and a lean body. I am living proof of that.

The bottom line to my story is that learning to control *ourselves* is the only way we will be able to achieve our weight loss goals, because often our environment is not under our control.

In Section 12, I will show you, in 7 Simple Steps, how to make permanent changes in your eating habits, including how to make junk food special again. So who said you can't have your cake and eat it too?

Section 6: More Weight Loss Mistakes

As I mentioned earlier, one of the biggest mistakes we make when trying to lose weight is trying to make too many changes in our lives at one time. Many weight loss programs tell us to make all those changes at once. In this section I will talk about three more common mistakes that sabotage countless weight loss efforts.

Mistake #1: Loss of focus

Although most of us start a weight loss program with a goal in mind, as the program progresses we lose focus on our objective and the benefits we will reap by sticking to the program. Instead we start focusing on the discomfort of exercising, and feelings of deprivation such as missing our favorite TV shows because we have to go to the gym, or not being able to eat whatever we want.

As you know, we are a "NOW" society; we want everything *now*. We don't want to wait. So, the immediate pleasure of eating what we want *now,* or watching our favorite TV shows *now* usually wins over the benefits we will enjoy in the future if we go through some minor discomfort *now*. We are torn between the urge on the one hand, to indulge in minor pleasures *now* and avoid minor discomforts *now*, and, on the other hand, the goal of achieving major benefits in the future by going through those minor discomforts *now*. Unfortunately, in most cases, the first option wins.

How to avoid making this mistake

You can avoid making the same mistake by creating a "trigger" to help you stay focused on your goal. What is a trigger? Have you ever heard a song that reminded you of a certain time in your life, or a certain place or person? The song is a "trigger" that brings back memories. Somehow, in your head, the song is linked with that certain place, person, or time in your life.

Here's how you can intentionally create a trigger to help you stay focused on your weight loss goal. Before you get started with any weight loss program, sit down in a quiet place and write down all the reasons why getting in shape and/or losing weight is important to you. How you are going to feel once you have achieved the body you want? How is getting fit going to affect your life and how other people see you? Keep writing all the benefits you hope to reap from getting in shape and/or losing weight. Don't be shy; write down as many as you can think of. No one but you needs to see this list.

Once you have completed the list, read it. As you do this, picture yourself already at your goal. How do you feel about yourself when you see yourself at the goal? How do other people feel about you? Maybe everybody who cares about you is proud — or even jealous! When you're at the peak of feeling great, do a small action, like pinching your thumb (or any other small action that can be easily done in public). Again, think about, and begin to feel, how great you'll look and feel when you have achieved your fitness goal, and pinch your thumb again. With your mind's eye, clearly see yourself at your fitness goal and keep pinching your thumb. Do this for at least for 10 minutes.

What you're trying to do is create a link between the everyday action of pinching your thumb and how you are going to feel when you have achieved your goal. It's the same concept as Ivan Pavlov's famous conditioning experiment. He got a dog to associate the ringing of a bell with the presence of food, so after a while the dog started salivating when it heard the bell, even when food was not present. We want to condition ourselves in the same way. Instead of the bell we'll use the pinching of our thumb (or whatever action you choose to use), and the automatic response we want is the feeling of well-being and accomplishment we'll feel when we achieve our fitness goals.

After you have created your trigger, practice it throughout the day. Keep practicing every day for one to two minutes, for at least 21 days straight. After that, the action of pinching your thumb will remind you of your fitness goals and how good you're going to feel when you have achieved them. As you start to apply the new eating habits into your life, you can use the trigger to help you get through cravings and stay focused on your fitness goals.

As a backup plan to help you stay focused, start another list of the negative effects you will experience if you continue with your current lifestyle habits. How are you going to look and feel one year from now if you continue the way you are, without making any lifestyle changes? How will your body look? How much might you weigh? How good or poor will your health be? How will other people see you? Picture yourself five years from now, 10 years from now, and 20 years from now — if you think you could live another 20 years with your current lifestyle. Don't leave any detail out. It may even help you to talk to people who didn't take care of their health when they were younger, and who now suffer because of it.

Take the two lists you created — the one you used to create your trigger, and the one that lists all the potentially negative effects of your current lifestyle — and put them aside. Look at both lists every weekend to remind yourself of the benefits you're working toward, and also the consequences of not sticking to your program. During your weight loss program, when you find yourself focusing on the discomforts you're enduring in order to achieve your goals, pull out the two lists and read them. Remind yourself that you have a simple choice: you can endure minor discomforts now and reap the health benefits they'll lead to in the future, or you can continue as you are, and run the risk of suffering major discomforts from diseases (diabetes, heart disease, hypertension, etc.) that will most likely develop from an unhealthy lifestyle. It's your choice. Knowing that, may motivate you to stick to your weight loss program.

Mistake #2: Following an incomplete weight loss program

As you might already know, misinformation in the weight loss field sabotages countless efforts to lose weight and get in shape. The biggest problem I find with most weight loss programs is that they offer only part of the solution to a weight problem. No matter how well we follow an "incomplete" weight loss program, any results we get will not be permanent, or even sustainable. For any weight loss program to be *complete*, it must include three things: some form of strength training, some form of aerobic activity, and it must not merely teach proper nutrition in terms of what to eat, and how to eat, but it should teach people how to make proper nutrition habitual. Any weight loss program that does not include those three things is doomed to fail from the start.

How many times have you seen aerobic machines like steppers and treadmills promoted as though they are the only things needed for losing weight and getting a fit body? If we were to follow that advice, we'd lose some weight initially. However, after a while the weight loss would stop.

Some aerobic equipment also offers a diet plan with it, so let's say we follow that diet and lose some more weight. Even then, the weight loss will stop after a while. Why? Because, when trying to lose weight by aerobics or aerobics and diet only, up to 25% of the weight that is lost is muscle. As we lose muscle mass, our metabolic rate slows down, and we all know what happens when our metabolic rate slows down. Weight loss stops unless we further reduce the calories that we take in. By doing some form of resistance training as we are losing weight, we ensure that our body will maintain the muscle, which will keep our metabolic rate higher, which is good for losing weight. This is only one example of what happens when a weight loss program does not incorporate strength training, aerobic activity, and proper nutrition.

How to avoid making this mistake

Make sure your weight loss program includes some form of strength training (free weights, Pilates, weight training machines, power yoga, etc.), some form of aerobics (treadmill, stepper, bike, walking outside, etc.), and proper nutrition (which you will learn in this book). The last and most important thing your weight loss program must have is a plan of action as to how you are going to incorporate all of the above into your life, without getting overwhelmed.

This book is part of your plan of action! In Section 12, I'll show you how to incorporate proper nutrition into your life in 7 Simple Steps. If you need help making exercise a habit in your life, I am currently working on a book that will help people develop the exercise habits, just like this one will help you develop the right eating habits. This book will be published sometime at the end of 2012. If you would like to be notified when my book on exercise is published please send an e-mail to **Stavros@LiveYourWayThin.com** and put "exercise book" in the subject line.

Mistake #3: Counting calories

This is the greatest mistake I see most diets and, unfortunately, most nutritionists make when trying to help their clients lose weight. There are two main problems with counting calories. First, it is very hard to keep up for life. Have you ever try to keep track of the calories you eat every day? I have, and I know is very hard, especially if you don't eat the same foods all the time. All the people that I know who have counted calories give up sooner or later, simply because it is too hard to do all the time. The second and biggest problem is the fact that we don't really know how many calories an individual really needs for optimum health. Yes, there are formulas that can help you estimate the number of calories you need, but I personally think those formulas are "off." The reason I first questioned those formulas is because I had read of many people who had robust health even though they were eating way under the recommended number of calories according to those formulas. I got really convinced when I learned to eat only when I was hungry, at least most of the time, and stopped eating when I had satisfied my hunger. After eating like that for over a year, I felt better than I had ever felt, and I found that I was eating 600 to 700 calories *less* per day than what the formulas said I should be eating. During the same period my workouts were going great and my strength was increasing, so I knew I wasn't undereating. If I was undereating, my strength and my feeling of well-being would be declining.

To figure out how many calories you need, you have to figure out your metabolic rate, which is determined by measuring the amount of oxygen your body uses. This varies with age, sex, habits, your diet, mental state, race, and many other factors. Scientists cannot really tell what the biological norm should be. "Normal" metabolism was determined by taking a mere statistical average metabolic rate of, for the most part, over-fed (especially over-protein-fed), over-stimulated human subjects. This does not make it a healthy metabolic rate; this is merely what the formulas that determine the number of calories you should have are based on. So the bottom line is, scientists don't really know how many calories you need for optimum health, they are only guessing, at best. Your body and only your body can tell you how much to eat; you just have to learn to listen to it.

How to avoid making this mistake
Learn to listen to your body. Your body will tell you when it needs food and when it does not. Your body will tell you when you have had enough food. Learn the signals your body gives you, you will not have to count calories.

Section 7: A Word on Detoxifying

There have been many books written about detoxifying and there are many products that claim to help you detoxify. First of all, you do not need to eat anything in order for your body to detoxify. Your body can detoxify all on its own, all we need to do is get out of its way and stop blocking the process. Here is how the process works. Every day, through the air we breathe, the liquids we drink, and the foods we eat, toxic substances enter our body and need to be eliminated. In addition, just the natural breakdown of food and the everyday functions of the body create waste matter that needs to be eliminated. What we need to do is ensure that the body's natural process of eliminating toxins and waste matter does not get interrupted or slowed down. What could slow down the elimination process? One thing is eating and digestion. If you are constantly eating and never give your body a break from food, the body can't do its job of eliminating toxins. The end result is that toxins come into the body at a much faster rate than they are eliminated, so they begin to accumulate in the system, which can create a host of health problems for the body. By following my 3 most important Eating Habits (eat only when hungry, eat slowly and mindfully, and stop eating when you have satisfied your hunger), you actually give your body more time to detoxify on a daily basis.

However, I still think it's a good idea to do a cleansing diet every three to four months. In the Greek Orthodox Church when we fast, we eat only fruits and vegetables; that is the kind of cleansing diet I recommend.

The cleansing diet

The best fruits for cleansing are oranges, grapefruit, grapes, and apples. The best vegetables are green, non-starchy vegetables like spinach, chicory, and romaine lettuce. Do not use any kind of dressing on your vegetables except perhaps some lemon juice.

If you're doing a fruit-only cleansing diet, eat only one type of fruit per meal, and eat only when you are hungry. You will find you will be getting hungry more often so you will be eating more often than when you're eating your normal foods. Most likely you will end up eating three to five times each day. If you want to eat vegetables too, eat them at a meal separately from fruit. So if you eat three meals each day, you can eat fruits at one meal and vegetables for the other two meals.

Do be careful, because the cleansing diet does not provide all the nutrients your body needs. My suggestion is not to stay on it for more than a week, though doing it even for just a day will have benefits.

Section 8:
The 3 Most Important Eating Habits
That Most Diets Don't Teach You

There are countless diets on the market today, each proclaiming they have the answer as to what foods you should eat and what foods you should avoid if you want to lose weight and improve your health. The high-protein diets say that if you simply cut carbs you will lose weight. The vegetarian diets proclaim that meat is the problem. The low-fat diets claim that fat is the problem. Then you have the everything in-between diets. Just as a side note, as far as weight loss is concerned, the proportion of protein, fat, and carbs in a diet has no effect on fat loss. If you eat more calories than what your body needs you will gain weight (fat), regardless of whether the extra calories came from fat, protein, or carbs. This is according to a study published in the Journal of the American Medical Association in January 2012.

The diet industry has been so busy debating the proportions of protein, fats and carbs in our diet, and how to "label" foods —healthy or unhealthy, fattening or non-fattening — they forgot the reasons why we are eating in the first place. Other very important questions that most diets have not pondered include: what is the best way to eat to aid digestion and increase satisfaction from food? Because the bottom line is, unless the food gets digested properly, it will not do us any good; as a matter of fact, improper digestion can be harmful to our health even if the food we ate was considered healthy. Another very important question is: when should we stop eating? And trust me when I tell you, trying to figure out how much to eat by counting calories is not a solution, because, as I explained earlier, we are not even sure how many calories one should eat in the first place. You body and only your body can really tell you when to eat, and when to stop eating. The key is to learn to pay attention to your body's signals.

In this section of the book I will teach you the 3 most important Eating Habits you can develop that will have the biggest effect on your health. The first and most important habit is to learn to *eat only when you are hungry* (at least most of the time), second, to learn to *eat slowly and mindfully*, and third, to learn to *stop eating when you have satisfied your hunger* (again, most of the time). Believe it or not, all 3 Eating Habits can be easily learned once you have learned to pay attention to your body. Notice there is no mention of the foods that you eat. I am not saying that what you eat does not play an important role in your weight and health; of course it does. What I am saying is that the reason you eat, how you eat, and when you stop eating is as important as what food you eat.

An experiment that supports the importance of these 3 habits

To show how important these 3 Eating Habits are to your weight and health, I did a very interesting experiment in October 2011. Before I started the experiment, I had a lipid profile done, measuring my cholesterol and triglycerides, I had my blood pressure done, and I weighed myself. I also kept track of my workouts, which for the duration of the experiment, I kept exactly the same.

For two months, Monday through Friday, I ate at fast-food restaurants only, mostly at McDonalds. I did not have their salads; I ate mostly cheeseburgers, Big Macs, Whoppers, and French fries. The only other thing I ate during the week was two servings of fruits or vegetables because I believe fruits and vegetables are essential to good health. On the weekends, I ate my normal diet, which included cookies, ice cream, soda, and many other junk foods.

During the week, when I was eating at fast-food restaurants, I ate according to the 3 Eating Habits. I ate only when I was hungry, I ate every meal slowly and mindfully, and I stopped eating when I had satisfied my hunger. Keep in mind, I only followed these 3 Eating Habits during the week. On the weekends I had no rules, so many times I did overeat and I did eat when I was not hungry.

So here are the results. At the end of two months of eating this way, my cholesterol went from 168 to 158, my triglycerides went from 57 down to 50, my blood pressure stayed the same at 113/68, and my weight went down 3 lbs, from 169 to 166. This goes to show you how important the 3 Eating Habits are. The point of this experiment was not to show that cheeseburgers and French fries are good or bad for you, but to show that if we eat the way nature intended, your body can deal with almost any food, whether it's considered healthy or unhealthy.

Here are the 3 most important eating habits you can develop, in more detail

Eating Habit #1
Eat only when you are genuinely hungry
What is the real purpose of eating? The real purpose of eating is *not* to entertain your mouth, although that is fine once in a while. It is *not* to increase your metabolic rate (one of the reasons they tell you to have breakfast), and it is *not* because you need to "stuff down" an emotion.

The real purpose of eating is to nourish your body, that is all. Eating for any other reason, no matter how you justify it, is harmful to your body. So the question is, how can you tell whether your body needs nourishment? Not by the clock. The only way to tell your body needs nourishment is through genuine hunger. The key is to learn what genuine hunger feels like so you can differentiate it from cravings. Unfortunately, the diet industry has taught people to eat by the clock and for reasons other than true hunger. For example, we are taught to eat breakfast whether we are hungry or not. They tell you breakfast is the most important meal of the day, but it is not. As a matter of fact, it might be the worst meal of the day. There is more on breakfast in a later section of this book. Some diets tell us we need to eat five to six meals throughout the day, regardless of whether we are actually hungry. The worst advice I have ever heard is to never let yourself go hungry because your body will think you are starving, so it slows your metabolic rate and tries to hold on to fat and burn your muscles. NOTHING will happen to you if you go hungry. As a matter of fact, the best thing you can do for your body is wait until you feel true hunger before you eat.

Here is a fact. Eating anything beyond what your body needs is harmful to your body, whether is considered healthy or unhealthy. Think about it, there's a reason why our body has a hunger mechanism, and I am sure it was not put there to be ignored. The only time you cannot go by hunger is if you are anorexic or you have Prader Willi Syndrome. Anorexics have lost the ability to tell when they are hungry and Prader Willi is a rare disorder that one of the effects is constant hunger, so either case they need specialized help beyond what this book was meant to provide. For the rest of us we can learn to pay attention to our hunger mechanism and eat only when genuinely hungry. Here are few more facts about hunger. Did you know that your eyesight, sense of smell, hearing, and focus improve when you are hungry? Keep in mind, we're talking about "hungry," not "starving." Many people use the word "starving" when they really mean "hungry." To starve is not to eat for days, not going hungry for a single day. Did you know the sense of taste improves with genuine hunger? You will get so much more enjoyment out of eating when you wait until you are truly hungry. Don't take my word for it, see for yourself!

Telling the difference between genuine hunger and cravings

Genuine hunger is a mouth and throat sensation just like thirst, and it derives from an actual physiological need for food. A craving is a counterfeit hunger, and it derives from a number of things including having a habitual snack after a meal, the smell of food, the sight of food, the arrival of a habitual meal time like breakfast, condiments and seasonings (for example: if you're not hungry, but you had a bite of a well-seasoned food, the seasoning can cause you to crave more food), the thought of food, or a conditioned response to stress, sadness, happiness, boredom, or any other emotion. Genuine hunger expresses the body's need for food. A craving expresses psychological wants and, as you know, sometimes what we want is not what we need. Unfortunately, many people give in to their wants and have to pay the consequences.   Genuine hunger comes instinctively, without the aid of some external factor. When you are genuinely hungry, you should have an empty feeling and a sense of low energy but not a feeling of weakness.   True hunger may also be accompanied by muscular contractions of the stomach. If you are truly hungry, you'll be willing to eat anything.

I love the way Dr. Herbert M. Shelton put it in his book, *The Hygienic System: Orthotropy*: "The hungry person is able to eat and relish a crust of dry bread; he who has only an appetite (craving) must have his food seasoned and spiced before he can enjoy it. Even a gourmand is able to enjoy a hearty meal if there is sufficient seasoning to whip up his jaded appetite and arouse his palsied taste. He would be far better off if he would await the arrival of hunger before eating."

I have heard many people complain that when they get hungry they get aches and pains or a lot of discomfort that disappears when they eat. This is not true hunger either. There is no pain or discomfort in genuine hunger. If you feel hungry and uncomfortable, you are having a craving. If you feel hungry and comfortable, then most likely you are truly hungry.

Food for many people has become like a drug, they eat so they can feel better or mask some other problem. Well, what happens to a drug addict who goes without a dose? The addict goes through a withdrawal. The same thing happens to food addicts. When they don't eat their customary meal or snack, they go through a withdrawal, and when they eat, the pain goes way, and the bad habit continues. So if your hunger is accompanied by some form of pain or discomfort, you are actually going through a withdrawal. Remember, genuine hunger is not accompanied by discomfort or pain. The best thing to do is to wait until the pain goes away. According to Dr. Herbert M. Shelton, "If we follow the rule to eat only when truly hungry, those people who are 'hungry' but weak and uncomfortable would fast until comfort and strength returned. Fasting would become one of the most common practices in our lives, at least, until we learn to live and eat to keep well and thus eliminate the need for fasting."

I know of people who claim they are always hungry. These people simply have not learned to distinguish the difference between genuine hunger and cravings or, even worse, a symptom of a disease.

The bottom line is, when you eat when you are genuinely hungry, your body is ready to receive food and digest it. When you eat for any other reason, no matter how healthful the food is, it is harmful to the body.

A word on preventive eating

Never engage in preventive eating, which is the habit of eating when you have time to — even if you're not hungry — because you don't think you'll have time to eat later. One of the unhealthiest things we can do, which contributes the most to weight gain, is eating when we're not physically hungry. If you eat when you're not hungry, most of the calories you consume at that time will be stored as fat. If you repeatedly find yourself in a situation where you have time to eat, but you're not hungry — but you eat anyway because you know you'll be hungry when you have no time to eat -— keep fruit or nuts with you. Snack on them when you get hungry — not before! Keep in mind though, even if you are hungry and you can't eat for few more hours, it's not the end of the world if you don't eat.

Hunger is *not* an emergency; as a matter of fact, it might be a good thing

Many of us are afraid to feel hunger. You can begin to lose this fear if you think of being hungry as a sign that your body is using its stored fat. If you keep supplying your body with fuel nonstop by eating all the time, why would your body use up its stored fuel (body fat)? Our bodies always prefer to use up fuel that just came in (the food we eat), rather than breaking down and using its stored fuel (body fat). We must give our bodies a chance to use up stored fuel if we want to lose weight.

But there is more to hunger than just burning excess fat. I have seen commercials for breakfast cereals that tell you hunger makes you lethargic and unable to focus, and that by eating you will focus better. The truth is the exact opposite. As I mentioned earlier, being hungry actually increases memory, learning, and the ability to focus. Studies, like one published in 2006 in the journal *Nature Neuroscience*, have shown that hunger actually can increase intelligence, happiness, and focus. When you stomach is emptied, it triggers the feeling of hunger by releasing a hormone called ghrelin. The same hormone has been found to increase learning, memory, and the ability to focus.

Forget for a second the studies and my personal experience, and let's look at this from a common sense perspective. If being hungry made us less focused, how would we have been able to find or capture our food in the days before grocery stores? Doesn't it make more sense that when we're hungry our focus and mental abilities would increase, so we can find food easier? Have you ever watched the National Geographic channel? Which lion looks more alert and focused — the hungry lion or the one that just ate? I personally have seen a huge difference in my alertness and ability to focus since I started letting myself get hungry before eating. I am 100% convinced that hunger affects our mental abilities in a very positive way.

Eat fewer times per day by eating only when you're hungry

Once you learn to eat only when you're hungry, you will find yourself eating only once or twice per day. You will find that most of the eating you were doing was out of habit, rather than genuine hunger.

Did you know that the three-meals-a-day custom is a modern tradition? Did you know that the Greek, Roman, and Persian armies at the period of their greatest power ate only one meal each day? That meal wasn't breakfast. It was dinner. Sometimes they did have a very light meal during the day, which was a biscuit and figs, or some kind of fruit. Those soldiers marched all day with heavy loads of armor on one meal per day and still had the energy to fight battles.

According to Dr. Felix Oswald, during the zenith period of Grecian and Roman civilization the rule was that a man who wanted to be healthy should content himself with one meal a day, and never eat till he had leisure time to digest after the meal. For more than a thousand years, one meal per day was the norm for most people around the Mediterranean.

England might have been one of the first countries to adopt the three-meals-per-day habit, which came along with the increased prosperity of the country. As a matter of fact, even today, the one thing that increases with wealth of the nation is that nation's food consumption. Dr. Herbert M. Shelton, in his book *The Hygienic System: Orthotrophy,* states: "as a general rule, that the quantity of food eaten in any country in all ages, has depended more upon their economic environment than upon their nutritional needs. Wealth and plenty have brought increased food consumption. In Ancient Rome these factors resulted in the eating of many meals a day, the eater taking an emetic immediately after finishing his gustatory enjoyment and then repairing to the vomitorium, after which he had another meal." We all know how Rome ended up.

A few months ago I was at a financial seminar, and one of the speakers talked about global opportunities for investing. What he said was very similar to Dr. Shelton's statement. He said that in countries with improving economies, like China, their consumption of food is increasing, so a good place to invest is in food production in those countries.

Eating only when you are genuinely hungry is the best habit you can develop for your weight and health.

You are most likely experiencing physical hunger when:
a. All food tastes good, including your least favorite foods
b. You have no doubt that you're hungry (If you're "not sure" whether you're hungry, then you're not)
c. You may feel "empty"
d. You may feel lightheaded
f. You may feel a loss of energy
g. You may feel a certainty that you must eat *now*
h. All you want to do is eat (If you feel like doing something other than eating, then you are not physically hungry)

You are most likely experiencing a craving when:
a. You weren't hungry until you saw or smelled food
b. You're searching your kitchen to find a food to satisfy a craving
c. You just want to suck on or chew something
d. You're feeling bored, angry, or anxious and you feel like eating something
e. You're thirsty
f. Your energy is low due to lack of sleep

Eating Habit #2
Chew your food well and eat slowly and mindfully
This habit alone can help you lose weight and aid your digestion. As you might already know, digestion begins in the mouth, by the mechanical process of chewing food. The benefit of chewing your food well is the fact that you break it down into smaller pieces so the digestive juices have more surface to work on. Also the saliva will begin to break down the starches in your food. Another benefit of chewing your food well is that you get to really taste what you eating. You will find that processed food will not taste as good because you will be able to taste all the additives in the food. You will begin to appreciate natural foods better when you really get to

taste them.

The benefit of eating slowly and mindfully is that you will end up eating less food.

Studies have shown that people who eat more slowly eat less than people who eat faster. There are a couple of reasons why most people eat less when they eat slowly. One reason is, by eating more slowly, you give your brain a chance to register that you are full. It takes up to 20 minutes for your brain to get the message that your stomach is full. The reason it takes that long is because the signal comes from the intestines, not the stomach, and it takes time for food to get to the intestines. Additionally, by eating slowly and more mindfully, you'll feel more satisfied by the end of the meal, so you'll be less likely to ask for seconds.

Let me tell you a story my friend Jim told me, which perfectly illustrates my point. Jim and his family had gone out to a restaurant to eat. That particular day, everybody was really hungry. Although the food was great, the service wasn't. First came the appetizers. After Jim and his family had finished their appetizers, the server took 20 minutes to bring their salads. After they had finished their salads, the server didn't bring their entrées for another 20 to 30 minutes.

Although everybody was very hungry when they first got to the restaurant, by the time the entrées came, everybody was full from having eaten only an appetizer and a salad. Usually, Jim said, he and his family could eat the appetizer, the salad, and the entrée with no problem. By simply waiting a little longer (even though it wasn't by choice), they felt full after having eaten less food. So you see, simply by eating more slowly, your brain has the chance to get the message that you had enough food and that you are satisfied, allowing you to eat less and lose weight.

Here's an exercise to try, which may help you to eat more slowly and mindfully. Eat three or four raisins, but take 10 to 20 minutes to eat them. Eat one at a time, and spend several minutes chewing patiently, holding the raisin in your mouth. Really try to taste all its flavors and notice all its textures before swallowing. I know this sounds a little ridiculous, but it's a great way to help you slow down when eating and also get more satisfaction out of each bite, which in turn will cause you to eat less. I recommend doing this exercise at least once each week; more if possible. If you want to get even more serious about eating mindfully, find a local Buddhist temple that practices mindful eating (which has been part of Buddhist teachings for centuries) and go to one of their events. If you live in the New York area, a great place to go to practice mindful eating is the Blue Cliff Monastery in Pine Bush, New York. Their website is www.bluecliffmonastery.org.

Here are few suggestions to help you develop this habit
1. Put down your fork between bites.
2. Be mindful of chewing your food. You can even count the number of times you chewed your food before swallowing. I recommend at least 20 times. While chewing, try to taste the food, of its spices and flavors.
3. If you're eating a sandwich, always put it down between bites.
4. Never do anything else while eating (watching TV, having a meeting, playing games, having a serious conversation, etc.). It takes your attention away from the meal and you will end up eating more than if you paid attention.
5. Try not to talk during a meal, if possible.

Eating Habit #3
Stop eating when you've satisfied your hunger
When do you know you've had enough food? For many of us, eating "enough" food means feeling stuffed to the point where we can hardly move. For others of us, it means we must eat all the food on our plate, no matter how our stomachs feel. Others of us feel we must unbuckle our belts at least one notch. There are many definitions we use to denote the "right" amount of food. If you want to lose weight, you have to make sure you have a realistic definition.

My definition of the "right" amount of food is when I have eaten enough to satisfy my hunger, but I feel I could eat a little bit more.

Keep in mind; it can take up to 20 minutes for your brain to get the message that you have eaten enough. That's why you should eat slowly and stop at a point where you feel you could eat a little bit more. Your stomach should not feel "stretched," and you should be able to take a brisk walk. If your stomach feels uncomfortable, you ate too much. Another way you can tell you had enough food is by the taste of the food. If you have developed Eating Habit #2 and you pay attention to the taste of the food, you will realize that the first bite always tastes the best. At some point, you will notice that the food doesn't taste as good as the first bite did. That is a sign that you have satisfied your hunger and that you should stop eating.

It's worth noting that the citizens of Okinawa, Japan practice something called *hara hachi bu*, which means they eat until they feel only 80% full. According to Dr. Bradley J. Willcox, Dr. Craig Willcox, and Dr. Makoto Sukuzi, authors of *The Okinawa Diet,* the island of Okinawa has the highest occurrence of centenarians and the longest life expectancies in the world. In addition, Okinawans have one of the lowest rates of disease, from cancer to cardiovascular disease.

One of the reasons for the Okinawans' long, healthy lives, besides their consumption of mostly fruits vegetables and fruits and their minimal consumption of meats, is the low-calorie diet they eat. Eating slowly is one way that anybody can begin to "cut calories." Because Okinawans stop eating when they feel 80% full, they eat fewer calories per day for their body weight than we do here in the States. It's believed that eating less causes your body to builds fewer free radicals (unstable molecules that damage vital body molecules such as tissues, DNA, etc., and cause disease). Free radicals are generated mainly through the metabolizing of food into energy, so the less you eat, the fewer free radicals you build up.

Once you have implemented these 3 Eating Habits, you will find yourself eating a lot less food than you used to. Although I don't believe in counting calories, if you calculate how many calories you eat once you've implemented these Eating Habits, don't be surprised if you eat less than the recommended calories for a person of your height and activity level. Listening to your body is a much better way to figure out how much to eat, rather than by following some formula that is based on averages.

Section 9: 4 More Eating Habits You Should Develop

In the previous section you learned about the 3 most important eating habits you can develop. They dealt with, when to eat, how to eat and when to stop eating. In this section we will cover 4 more very important eating habits that deal with what foods to eat and what foods to cut down on. This can be a very confusing subject. There are so many contradicting opinions on what foods we should be eat and what foods we should be avoiding, it's hard to know exactly what we should be eating. Even I, during my first 10 years in the fitness field, was confused trying to figure out the best way to eat, not just for weight loss, but also for optimum health. And you can't always trust studies. If you look hard enough, you can find studies to prove almost anything you want. There are studies that show that high protein diets are a great way to lose weight, and there are studies to show that high protein diets are very bad for your health, just to give you one example.

To try to get closer to the answer of which foods are best, I decided to look at cultures in which people live very long, healthy lives. That's when I started looking at "Blue Zones" (author Dan Buettner's name for geographic areas where people live long and healthy lives) and realized that the typical Greek island diet, on which I was raised, is considered one of the healthiest diets on earth. As a matter of fact, the Greek island of Ikaria is considered one of the "Blue Zones." The diet and lifestyle on Ikaria is very similar to the way I was brought up on my home island of Evia. According to Dan Buettner, author of *The Blue Zones*, Ikaria is home to the highest percentage of people who live past 90 years of age. This is when I finally started coming up with answers as far as what would be the best way to eat.

I do realize that each of us is not able to live the same lifestyle as people who live on Ikaria or in other Blue Zones, but we can incorporate a lot of their eating habits into our lives. By looking at studies as well as by looking at how people live in those healthy regions around the earth and using some common sense, I identified 7 Eating Habits that I consider the most important for our weight and health. In the previous section I covered 3 of the 7 Eating Habits. In this section I will cover the 4 remaining Eating Habits that deal with the foods we should be eating and foods we should be cutting down on.

Although there is more to proper nutrition than the 7 Eating Habits I cover in this book, if you make these habits part of your lifestyle, not only will you lose all the weight you want, you'll also be much better off, health-wise, than you were before. Now let's take a look at the remaining 4 Eating Habits you should be developing.

Eating Habit #4
Make junk food special
Have junk food on weekends and special occasions *only*. Junk food is here to stay, but with this habit, you can learn to live with it and still lose weight. Don't worry about how you'll be able to eliminate junk food from your weekdays. There's a very simple way to achieve this, which I will describe in Section 12.

Eating Habit #5
Eat at least 5 servings of vegetables and fruits per day, preferably more
Vegetables and fruits are excellent sources of vitamins, antioxidants, phytochemicals, minerals, and fiber. There is

abundant evidence to support the notion that high intake of vegetables and fruits greatly reduces the risk of developing cancer, cardiovascular disease, inflammatory diseases, and many other chronic diseases. A diet high in fruits and vegetables is a must if you want to greatly improve your chances of living a long and healthy life. A review of 200 epidemiological studies found that people who consumed diets high in fruits and vegetables had a 50 percent lower cancer risk, compared to people who ate only a few fruits and vegetables. My suggestion is to try to eat more of the servings from vegetables, rather than fruits.

Eating Habit #6
Eat at least one serving of beans/legumes at least 5 days each week, every day if possible

Why eat beans/legumes? For one thing, beans have been shown to have a cholesterol-lowering effect. Beans have a low glycemic index and, because of that, they play a positive role in preventing diabetes and obesity. In addition, beans appear to protect against cancer due to the phytochemicals and antinutrients they contain. There are great-tasting bean recipes in the Members' Section of my website, www.liveyourwaythin.com. Membership is free.

Eating Habit #7
Don't eat more than 5 servings of meat or poultry each week

Most people have a very hard time following this rule. Many people believe it's essential to have some form of meat every day. This can't be further from the truth, but there was once a time when I believed it too. At one point I was certified to teach a diet similar to the Zone Diet. Over the years, and after countless hours of reading nutritional studies and reports, I changed my mind. The one study that convinced me to eat less meat was the China Project, a study jointly conducted by researchers from Oxford University, Cornell University, and academic institutions in China. The China Project showed that, as consumption of animal products increased, so did cancer and heart disease. Animal products are essential to the diet, but not in large quantities. For more information on the China

Project, go to *www.nutrition.cornell.edu/ChinaProject/*. As far as where you are going to get your protein from, don't worry about it. Although protein is an essential nutrient, the amount we need has been greatly exaggerated. In addition they have made us believe that meat is the only source. Vegetable, beans, and nuts all have protein, and although they might be missing one of the nine essential amino acids, most people eat enough variety to get the missing amino acid from another foods. Think about this. What do the largest land animals like the elephants and rhinos eat? Grass and leaves not meat and somehow are able to build all that muscle. In addition to that, I realized that when I lived in Greece, on average most people ate meat (including chicken) only once or twice per week. We ate fish once a week, and the rest of the time we ate vegetarian dishes, many of which included beans. Although we ate meat and fish only three times per week on average, nobody had a protein deficiency.

There's more...
Of course there's more to a health-enhancing diet than the 7 Eating Habits, but I think these are the most important habits you should develop, which will have the biggest effect on your weight and health. I suggest that you start your weight loss program by incorporating these 7 Eating Habits into your life and, once they have become second nature, you can make even more improvements in your diet. There are plenty of ideas on my website, www.liveyourwaythin.com, or my Olympus fan page on Facebook.

These 7 Eating Habits will not do you any good unless they become a part of your life. You can't just follow them once in a while and expect to get results. In Section 12, I will show you, through 7 Simple Steps, how to make these 7 Eating Habits *your* eating habits.

Section 10:
A Few More Things You Need to Know About Eating

When is the best time to eat your main meal?
The answer might surprise you. The best time to eat your main meal of the day is at a time when you can rest afterwards. In Greece we had our main meal at lunch, but we got a three-hour break afterwards to relax and take a nap. I strongly believe the main meal in America should be eaten in the evening after work due to the fact that we don't have leisure time during the day like they do in Greece.

Here's why it's important to rest after a large meal. Emotions and moods greatly influence the secretion of digestive juices. People in a good mood have better secretion of digestive juices. Negative emotions like worry, fear, anger etc., all influence digestion in a bad way. They stop the secretion of digestive juices and the rhythmic motions of the stomach, as well as the secretion of saliva.

Another factor that affects digestion is the availability of blood. For digestion to proceed normally, blood has to rush to the digestive organs in large quantities. For that to happen, blood vessels that supply organs not essential to digestion constrict to force blood to the organs required for digestion. If, after a main meal, you go right to work (be it physical or mental), your brain and muscles will also need blood to function correctly. That means the blood vessels supplying the brain and muscles will not constrict, so additional blood will not rush to the digestive organs to help with digestion. Therefore, digestion gets compromised.

Have you noticed how you feel after eating a main meal? Don't you feel like taking a nap? Well, that's normal. Most of your energy has to go toward digesting the food you just ate. That is why in all the cultures in which people eat their main meal at lunch, there is a long break after eating. Since those of us in America can't take long lunch breaks complete with a nap, the best thing to do is eat a very light lunch (only if you are hungry, of course) and eat our main meal at night, when the full attention of the body can go toward digestion.

Look at animals in nature. After a lion eats, it rests; it doesn't run around. Animals instinctively know what to do. Humans, unfortunately, have lost that instinct, but we can get it back by paying closer attention to our bodies.

A word on breakfast

Definitely not the most important meal of the day. Possibly the worst meal of the day! Just in case all of the above facts have not convinced you that you should not eat a main meal in the morning, let me debunk few myths about breakfast.

The main reasons I hear for eating breakfast are: 1) Breakfast gives you energy to get through your morning, 2) Eating breakfast increases your metabolic rate. Let me first tackle #2. The only reason it increases your metabolic rate is because of the thermic effect of food. Basically, your metabolic rate increases to burn off the food you just ate. In addition, I have a question for all those nutritionists: what is wrong with a slow metabolic rate, health-wise? I can answer that question: NOTHING! As a matter of fact, you *want* a slower metabolic rate because that means you can survive on less food and take advantage of the host of health benefits that come from eating less food

Now for the claim that breakfast supplies energy to get you through the morning. In order for food to give you any energy, it has to first be digested, go through the intestine and be absorbed by the body. The process can take more than 6 hours! So you see, the morning meal, unless it's fruit, which can be digested quickly, can't provide energy for the day. As a matter of fact, it takes energy away from your day, because your body now requires energy for digesting breakfast.

Another question: if breakfast is so important, why are most people are not hungry in the morning? I'm willing to bet that most people who think they're hungry in the morning are just feeling a habitual hunger, more like a craving. Just in case you think I am crazy, investigate all the healthy cultures around the world and you'll find that breakfast is nonexistent or very small. In Greece, on the island I lived on, most adults did not have breakfast. They usually had a Greek coffee and sometimes a biscuit. The evening meal was larger, because it had time to be fully digested and absorbed by the body overnight. That was the meal that supplied the energy for the next day. The best thing to do is try it yourself. Skip breakfast for few weeks and see what happens.

Stavros Mastrogiannis

Section 11: Your Attitude Will Determine Your Success

The one thing that will have the biggest effect on whether or not you achieve your weight loss goal is your attitude. You must have a winning attitude. Many people, although they would like to lose weight and get in shape, deep down don't truly believe they can do it. One of the reasons they think that is because they have failed so many times before, they have trained themselves to expect failure. As the saying goes, "Whether you think you can or you think you can't, you are right."

So, what is a winning attitude? Whether you realize it or not, we all talk to ourselves. Sometimes the talk is negative and sometimes it's positive. People who don't have a winning attitude talk to themselves like this: *I can't control myself. If I see a piece of chocolate, I must have it. What's the point of losing weight; I'm only going to gain it all back. I can't lose weight, I'm genetically programmed to be overweight. I'm fine compared to everybody else. I don't have time to exercise. I can't stop eating. I can't do this.*

You see, the focus is on why we *can't* do what we need to do and also why we shouldn't even bother. A person who truly believes any of the statements above will never be able to lose weight, and here is why: Your brain is like a search engine. You put your question in, it comes up with answers. The problem is that it will not reject any questions or statement and tell you that is not true, it will simply come up with answers. If you say to yourself, "I can't lose weight," you brain finds reasons to support that statement.

This is not helpful to you, so what can you do about it? Ask a better question, or make a better statement. The best questions to ask are "How" questions. So, instead of saying to yourself, "I can't lose weight" change that to, "How can I lose weight?," or "What can I do today to move closer to my weight loss goal?" These are much better questions because now your brain will start searching for things you can do today to help you move closer to your goal.

Having a winning attitude will help tremendously to keep you positive as you are going through the process of eliminating bad eating habits and adopting new ones. As you might already know, there will be times when you will fall off the plan, and that's normal. Having a winning attitude will help you get back on the plan. All my successful clients fell off the plan at some point, but they got right back on it. The difference between people who succeed and people who do not succeed, is that people who succeed learn from any setbacks, shrug it off and move on. People who are not successful dwell on setbacks, justify their failure, and quit. Let me tell you ahead of time, you will have setbacks; they're part of the learning curve. Just learn from your setbacks and move on.

Section 12:
How to Change to the New Way of Eating
Without Getting Overwhelmed

Changing eating habits is hard, at least that's what most people think. But the only reason changing eating habits is hard is because of the way most diets want you to change them, which is all at once. Changing eating habits actually is not as hard as most people think, if you do it the right way. So what is the right way? Well, let's think about this.

Over the years we all have developed routines that require very little active thinking on our part. For example, how many times have you driven to work, and when you got there, you found that you remembered hardly anything about the drive. It has become such a routine, it's almost like you are on autopilot. As long as we stay within our daily routines, we are in our comfort zone.

Do you remember a time that you started a new, unfamiliar task? I am sure it felt uncomfortable and required a lot of thinking. The new task moved you outside your comfort zone and until it became familiar and the task moved within your comfort zone. Keep in mind, the more new tasks you try to do at the same time, the further outside your comfort zone you move, and the more uncomfortable you become. Most people can tolerate small amounts of discomfort for a longer period, than they can tolerate large amount of discomfort, regardless of the benefits.

Confucius, a Chinese philosopher, said it best: "A journey of a thousand miles begins with a single step." The journey to a lean and healthy body begins with changing a single habit.

If you had to take a journey of a thousand miles and you focused on the thousand miles you must travel, it would overwhelm you, but if you focus on putting one foot in front of the other the journey would seem more manageable. It's the same thing with losing weight and getting in shape. To do those things, most people must change a number of eating and activity habits. If you look at all the habits you must change, that alone can overwhelm you. But, if you focus on changing one single habit at a time, the task becomes much more manageable.

By changing one habit at a time, you keep the discomfort low, which makes it much easier to tolerate it, which will greatly increase your chances of sticking with the new action long enough to make it a habit and part of your comfort zone. It takes around three to four weeks for a new task to become familiar, and it would take over six months for a familiar new task to become a habit.

A few more things before you start
It would be a good idea, but not necessary, if you can, to do three to six day of the cleansing diet I recommend in Section 7 before you begin changing your eating habits. There are two main reasons I recommend this. First, the obvious reason of cleansing your body of toxins and waste matter that has accumulated over the years. The second reason is, the discipline of the cleansing diet will strengthen your will, which it will make changing your eating habits so much easier. There is one more side benefit. For many people, food is like a drug, and just like a drug addict goes through a withdrawal, so does a food addict. Some people, when they start eating only when they are hungry, go through a period of minor headaches and other minor discomforts. By doing the cleansing diet first, you get those minor pains out of the way, so it makes it

easier to incorporate the first Eating Rule into your life.

A word of caution

As I have said, the biggest mistake you can make when trying to change your eating habits is to try to make many changes at once. Regardless of any results you achieve, you will get overwhelmed and quit. So please follow the upcoming 7 Simple Steps slowly and at your own pace. Each of the 7 Simple Steps outlined in this section will help you forge new eating habits in a meaningful, lasting way. Each step is designed to build upon the previous one, so please don't skip any steps unless the step you're working on asks you to do something you already do. For example, if the goal of a particular step is to get you to eat at least 5 servings of fruits and vegetables per day and you already do that, just skip that step and move to the next one.

Further help

I have created easy-to-use booklets that help track your progress at adapting each of the 7 Eating Habits into your life. You can purchase them on my website, www.liveyourwaythin.com.

A word about weekends

It's very important that you give yourself a break from all the new eating habits you are trying to develop. Sometimes I see people get so excited about losing weight, they want to work on all 7 Eating Habits every day. However, I've found over the years that people who are too strict burn themselves out. You must have one or two days each week when you can completely relax. Over time, you'll find that you're eating better, even on the weekends. If it happens, that's fine, but let it happen naturally. And, knowing you're allowed to eat what you want on the weekends will make it much easier to control yourself during the week. It's a way to make weekends even more special!

Prerequisites

Before you start on Step 1, you must do two things. First, you must develop a trigger that will remind you why you want to lose weight and get in shape. Having a strong trigger will be a big help in fighting off cravings as you go through each step. See Section 6 for detailed instructions on developing a trigger. Second, write the following question on a 3 x 5 card and place it on the bathroom mirror where you can read it every day. "What small action can I take today that would move me closer to my weight loss goal?" This question will train your brain to start looking for ways to help you achieve your weight loss goal.

The 7 Simple Steps To Permanent Weight Loss

STEP 1
Objective: Apply Eating Habit #1 *(Eat only when you are genuinely hungry)* Monday through Friday.
The first Eating Habit is the most important. Make sure you are clear about the difference between genuine hunger and cravings. If not, reread Eating Habit #1 in Section 8.

From now on, Monday through Friday (Friday until 5 pm; after 5 pm is part of the weekend), you will not eat unless you are genuinely hungry. Don't give yourself a choice. This is a rule you must follow, from now on. So from now on Monday through Friday (Friday until 5 pm), before you eat anything you must ask yourself, "Am I hungry?" If the answer is "no," or "not really," or if you're not sure, then don't eat. Eat only if you're absolutely positive that you are genuinely hungry. You don't have to apply this habit on the weekends, but don't go out of your way to break it, either.

Tips: I realize applying this habit might be hard for some people, especially those of us who are prone to cravings, or who turn to food for comfort after a long, stressful day. The secret of breaking those bad habits is to give yourself no choice. Let's say it's Monday and you've just had dinner and you're craving something sweet. If you sit and dwell on the craving, sooner or later you will find a way to justify why it's OK to have it, and you will give in. Instead what you want to do is remind yourself that is Monday and you have no choice. Tell yourself, "I am not hungry so I am not going to eat. What else can I do instead of eating?" You will be amazed how fast the craving goes away when you don't dwell on it. Here are some of the solutions my clients have come up with to deal with their cravings: surf the web, play games on their cell phones, read a book, take a walk, or call a friend. If you come up with a unique way of replacing stress eating with a more constructive activity, please let me know. You can e-mail me at stavros@liveyourwaythin.com.

By giving yourself no choice, and then choosing something else to do, other than eating, you will train yourself to eating only when hungry and sooner or later it will become automatic. As far as the weekends go, you will find that over time you will be eating only when you hungry at least most of the time.

When to move to the next step
Move to the next step only when you've had a week in which you applied Eating Habit #1 perfectly. In other words, a week during which you only ate because you were hungry Monday through Friday (Friday until 5 pm). However, even if you have completed a perfect week, you don't have to move to the next step until you feel ready. Take as much time as you like at each step. In fact, you're better off taking extra time at each step to make sure you're very comfortable with the new Eating Habit, rather than trying to move through the steps too quickly, before you've truly established the new Eating Habit.

STEP 2
Objective: Develop Eating Habit #2 (*Chew your food well and eat slowly and mindfully*) Monday through Friday (Friday until 5 pm). If you're not sure if you ate slowly and mindfully, you didn't.

Tip: Don't pre-cut your food. Cut one piece at a time and put down your knife and fork between bites. If you're eating a sandwich, put it down between bites. Chew a bite of food at least 20 times before swallowing (this is also good for digestion). Pay attention to the flavors and textures of the food you're eating.   For more information on this Eating Habit, go back to Section 8 and review it.

When to move to the next step
Move to the next step only when you've had a week in which you applied Eating Habit #2 perfectly. In other words, a week during which you ate every meal or snack Monday through Friday (Friday until 5 pm) slowly, mindfully, and chewing every bite really well. However, even if you have completed a perfect week, you don't have to move to the next step until you feel ready. Take as much time as you like at each step. In fact, you're better off taking extra time at each step to make sure you're very comfortable with the new Eating Habit, rather than trying to move through the steps too quickly, before you've truly established the new Eating Habit.

STEP 3
Objective: Develop Eating Habit #3 *(Stop eating when you've satisfied your hunger)* Monday through Friday (Friday until 5 pm). Review this Eating Habit in Section 8 to know exactly what the "right" amount of food is, and how to know when you've had enough.

Tip: Remember, it takes about 20 minutes for your brain to get the message that you are full. Stop eating at a point at which you feel you could eat more.

I would like to tell you a story one of my friends told me. He worked at a restaurant, and one day he was so busy, he didn't get a chance to eat until late afternoon. By that point he was really hungry, so he made himself a big bowl of pasta. He had only six bites before the phone rang. Although he was still hungry, he had to take the call. He stayed on the phone for 30 minutes and, when he went back to finish his meal, he realized he was no longer hungry. Usually he ate a whole bowl of pasta before he felt satisfied — and also stuffed — but on this particular day he had only six bites and felt he was satisfied, without that stuffed feeling. His story perfectly illustrates my point; if you eat slowly, and stop eating at a point at which you feel you could eat more, you'll find that you feel perfectly satisfied, even though you've eaten less food than you might have eaten if you'd eaten at a faster rate.

When to move to the next step

Move to the next step only when you've had a week in which you applied Eating Habit #3 perfectly. In other words, a week during which, Monday through Friday (Friday until 5 pm), you stopped eating every meal at a point at which you had satisfied your hunger but were not stuffed. However, even if you have completed a perfect week, you don't have to move to the next step until you feel ready. Take as much time as you like at each step. In fact, you're better off taking extra time at each step to make sure you're very comfortable with the new Eating Habit, rather than trying to move through the steps too quickly, before you've truly established the new Eating Habit.

Review

By this time, you should be eating only when you are physically hungry; eating every meal and snack slowly and mindfully and chewing every bite at least 20 times; and you should be able to stop eating at a point where you still feel slightly hungry, but satisfied. You should be able to do all of these things perfectly, Monday through Friday of every week.

By this point, you should be losing weight. If you aren't, you may not be applying the Eating Habits as well as you think you are. Even if you're losing weight at a very good rate (one to two lbs. per week), don't stop here. Take a one-to-two-week break before moving on, to continue practicing Simple Steps 1 – 3 and make sure the first three Eating Habits are part of your life and almost automatic. Then move on to the next step.

The following Simple Steps will help you implement the remaining 4 Eating Habits, which have to do with *what* you eat. These Eating Habits might help you speed up your weight loss a little bit more, but the main reason you want to incorporate them into your life is because they will have a big impact on improving your health. Remember, although losing weight and having a nice-looking body are great, enjoying good health and lowering your chances of developing deadly diseases is even better.

STEP 4

Objective: Develop Eating Habit #4 *(Make junk food special)* by eating junk food only on the weekends. From now on, you will have no junk food from Monday morning through 5 pm Friday. Because Friday nights are often considered part of the weekend, many people have a difficult time not having any junk food on Friday night. My rule is, it's OK to have one serving of junk food on Friday after 5 p.m., if you really feel you have to have it.

You can enjoy junk food guilt-free on the weekends. However, if a holiday or special occasion such as an anniversary, or if your own birthday falls on a weekday, it's OK to have some junk food. After all, we want to make junk food special, so you should be able to have it on special days. Predetermine what special occasions and holidays you can break this habit on.

If you feel you need more help dealing with the desire to eat junk food, I'm working on a book specifically about junk food, *Let's Make Junk Food Special Again*, which will be available in 2013.

Wine and beer

On the days when you're not supposed to have junk food, it's OK to have one small glass of wine or one bottle of beer if you really want to. More than one wine or beer is considered junk food, so you will be breaking the rule.

Tip: Do not remove junk food from your home. As I said in Section 5, you want to learn to control yourself, not your environment. If you have a strong craving, just remind yourself that you have no choice, and that you can indulge in the junk food you're craving the next day, when you can have it without feeling guilty. This is the time to use your trigger to remind yourself of your goals of a thinner body and increased health. Remember, dwelling on a craving gives it power over you. If you give yourself no choice, the craving loses its power.

When to move to the next step

When you have completed at least two weeks in a row of not having any junk food Monday morning through 5 p.m. Friday, you are ready to move to the next step. Remember, if you don't feel quite ready to move on, it's OK to stay at this step until you feel you have fully implemented this Eating Habit.

STEP 5

Objective: Develop Eating Habit #5 (Eat at least 5 servings of vegetables and fruits per day, preferably more)

Tip #1: Make a habit of having a good-sized salad before you eat dinner. The best dressing is olive oil and vinegar, but if you're going to have a creamy dressing, keep it on the side and dip your bare fork in it before you take a bite of your salad. Having a salad first will do two things: It will ensure that you get at least two servings of vegetables, plus it will curb your appetite a little so you will not overeat during dinner. Make sure your dinner also includes at least one vegetable.

You can get more fruits and vegetables into your day by carrying baby carrots, celery, or some kind of fruit with you to snack on if you get hungry. The key to getting more fruits and vegetables into your diet is to make them more available. You will find some delicious veggie recipes in Section 16 of this book.

Tip #2: Always make sure you have your favorite fruits available at work and at home. If you like a fruit that needs peeling or cutting, such as watermelon, cantaloupe, honeydew, etc. I suggest peeling and cutting it the night before, and placing it in a container to take it with you to work.

STEP 6

Objective: Develop Eating Habit #6 *(Eat at least one serving of beans/legumes at least 5 days each week, every day if possible)*

Tips: A serving of beans is ½ cup. Beans are one of the few foods whose nutritional value improves with the canning process, so canned beans are OK to use. Just make sure you rinse them, and try to select beans with low sodium. I have included a few easy-to-make bean recipes in Section 16 of this book. For more recipes, go to the Members' Section of my website, www.liveyourwaythin.com. Membership is free.

When to move to the next step
Move to the next step when you have completed at least two weeks of eating at least one serving of beans, 5 days each week.

STEP 7

Objective: Develop Eating Habit #7 *(Don't eat more than 5 servings of meat or poultry per week, preferably less)*
Tip: A serving of meat is the size and thickness of your palm. Many people complain that they don't feel satisfied unless they eat some kind of meat at every meal. I suggest replacing some of your meat dishes with beans or fish. Either one will satisfy you as well as meat. If you are having a vegetarian dish, put some olive oil on it. Oleic acid, a fatty acid found in olive oil and other unsaturated fats, satisfies hunger just like meat does.

Where to go from here

If you stick with everything you learn in these 7 Simple Steps, you should be able to keep off all the weight you lose. If you have not yet achieved your weight loss goal, as long as you stick with the 7 Eating Habits — and, of course, keep exercising — you'll keep losing weight until your body gets to the weight it was meant to be. If you're interested in making further improvements in your diet, become a member of my website at www.liveyourwaythin.com and you'll receive updates on the latest developments in diet and exercise. Membership is free.

Section 13:
Motivational Tips to Help you
With the Transition to the New Habits

Tip #1: Change your success indicator

To stay motivated, especially in the beginning when the weight might not be coming off as fast as you would like it to, you can keep yourself from getting discouraged by changing your success indicator.

Let me explain what I mean by that. Most of us, when we're trying to lose weight, use the scale as our success indicator. In other words, we weigh ourselves every week to see if the scale shows a lower number (which makes us feel successful) or a higher number (which makes us feel defeated). We can avoid motivation-destroying negative feelings by focusing not on the weight, but on the actions we're supposed to take in our weight loss program.

Let's say you are working on Step One (Developing the habit of eating only when hungry Monday through Friday). Additionally, you have a goal of doing three aerobic workouts and two strength training workouts that week. If you did all that, you had a successful week, *even if the number on the scale did not change.*

Nothing good comes out of using your weight as your success indicator. One problem with using weight as your success indicator is that sometimes you can do everything right, eat the perfect diet, do all your exercises, and the scale still doesn't move. This can happen for a multitude of reasons — eating salty food or a large meal before a weigh-in; for women, accumulated water weight during a menstrual cycle; or any number of other reasons. That's why it's more realistic and encouraging to focus on the habits you must develop in order to lose the weight you want.

So, at each step, make your success indicator the actions that you're asked to take. If you succeed in completing those actions, you had a successful week. Don't worry about the weight. If you follow the simple directions at each step, it's only a matter of time before the weight starts coming off.

Tip #2: Focus on the inspiration, not the challenge

The reason many people quit their efforts to lose weight and get in shape is because they focus too much on everything they must do in order to achieve the results they want. That can be overwhelming for most people. Instead, focus on how good it's going to feel when you have lost all the weight you want. To help you do that, do the following exercise: Write down at least 10 reasons why you what to lose weight and get in shape. Then write a short paragraph about how you are going to feel when you have lost the weight, and how others might react when they see you have lost the weight. How good would that feel? Be as descriptive as you can. Take a few minutes to read that paragraph to yourself every morning. This will help you stay focused on the reasons why you want to lose weight. Focus on what inspires you to lose weight, not what obstacles are in your way. I do this exercise myself, to help myself stay focused on my objectives in life. I highly recommend it.

Section 14: More Nutritional Advice

About whole grains
Whole grains do play an important role in health, but overeating them could contribute to obesity and weight gain. If you're going to have grain products like bread, bagels, cereals, etc., I recommend that you choose whole grain products. I don't have any specific recommendation on how many servings of whole grains one should have; one or two servings per day might not be a bad idea.

About dairy products
Dairy foods do have their benefits, especially fermented dairy foods such as yogurt, cottage cheese, and kefir. These fermented foods contain probiotics that are beneficial to our health. Though I don't think we need to drink milk as adults, I do recommend that people eat at least one serving of a fermented dairy product every day, or at least most days of the week. Although they are not well understood yet, probiotics play an important role in overall health, including the health of your gastrointestinal track and your immune system.

How much water should we drink?

I've heard different numbers as to how many glasses of water one should drink each day. In truth, the answer depends on what types of foods you consume. If your diet is made up of foods that have a high water content, like fruits and vegetables, and you don't eat a high amount of salt, you may be able to drink only three or four glasses of water each day. But if you eat a typical American diet high in meats, salt, and highly processed foods and low in fruits and vegetables, you might need to drink eight to 10 glasses of water per day. Of course, if you're very active, especially aerobically, drink more water.

I recommend that you drink at least six to eight glasses of water per day, more if you are very active, especially in hot weather. When you've established all of the 7 Eating Habits, you'll be eating foods with a higher water content, and can cut your water consumption to five to six glasses of water per day.

Although minimizing the use of salt is ideal, if you're eating a diet high in salt, I recommend that you drink at least eight to 10 glasses of water per day, more if you are active.

About artificial sweeteners

I don't recommend artificial sweeteners. Studies like one done in 1997 by J.H. Lavin, S.J. French, and N.W. Read, at the Centre for Human Nutrition, Northern General Hospital, Sheffield, U.K. suggest that people who use artificial sweeteners like aspartame make up for the calories they didn't consume due to the artificial sweetener, by eating more calories later. I have not seen a study that showed substituting sugar with artificial sweeteners made any difference in people's weight. The best thing to do is do cut down the amount of sugary beverages or foods you consume overall. If you're going to have a sweet treat, make sure it contains real sugar, not a substitute. We don't yet know all the effects artificial sweeteners can have on the body.

About coffee

If you're going to drink coffee, have it before noon and try not to have more than two cups per day. Drinking coffee later in the day will interfere with your sleep. Even if it doesn't keep you up at night, coffee does make you a light sleeper and it will affect the quality of sleep negatively. Not sleeping well or not sleeping enough has been shown to increase appetite the next day.

About weight loss drugs

Remember, to lose weight permanently you need to make permanent changes in your diet and exercise habits. Even if you found a drug that could really help you lose weight, you'd need to stay on it forever if you wanted to keep the weight off forever. The minute you went off the drug, the weight would come back.

All the weight loss drugs I'm aware of have side effects and were not meant for long-term use. How many times have you heard of some miracle new weight loss drug, only to hear about the drug's terrible side effects a few months later? Remember, the root causes of your weight problem are your dietary and exercise habits. Weight loss drugs only mask those problems; they don't fix anything. If you want to fix your weight loss problem forever, you must change the habits that made you overweight in the first place.

About dietary fats

Dietary fat isn't a problem if you develop the first three Eating Habits from this book. As long as you've made it a habit to eat only when you're hungry, to eat slowly and mindfully, and eat "just enough" food, even if you eat something that contains a considerable amount of fat, you'll find that you satisfy your hunger sooner, and you won't eat as much. It will also take you longer to get hungry again.

I can give you a personal example. If I have a salad for lunch (no meat, just vegetables) tossed with a little bit of olive oil and vinegar, I get hungry again after four or five hours, but if I have a slice of pizza for lunch I can go for at least seven hours before I get hungry again. The extra fat in the pizza satisfies my hunger for a much longer period.

The only fats I recommend avoiding are trans fats. Saturated fats, although you do want to limit them, are not as bad as trans fats. Besides, you'll cut down on your consumption of saturated fats naturally once you apply Eating Habit #7 (Don't eat more than 5 servings of meat or poultry each week).

Olive oil and flaxseed oil are the best fats. When making a salad or cooking a vegetarian meal, don't be afraid to use olive oil. Most of the Greek vegetarian dishes I was raised on had plenty of olive oil in them. Just make sure you eat only when you are hungry, eat slowly and mindfully, and stop eating when you have satisfied your hunger.

Section 15: A Few Words on Exercise

Although this book is about how to improve your diet so you can lose weight and improve your health, I want to make sure you realize that exercise plays a very important role in weight loss and health as well. The two forms of exercise you should include in your weight loss program are some form of strength training and some form of aerobic activity.

Why strength train?
Did you know that the average adult over the age of 25 loses four pounds of muscle every 10 years? That happens because the body does not like waste. At all times, it tries to conserve energy and get rid of anything it doesn't need, like extra muscle that it doesn't use. Since most people don't use their muscles for strenuous work on a regular basis, the body gets rid of the muscle it doesn't need.

Also, muscles themselves conserve energy by only utilizing the smallest number of fibers needed to complete a task. Let me explain. A muscle, depending on its size, is made up of hundreds of thousands of muscle fibers. The fibers are the units that contract and produce the power. If you don't need a lot of power, your muscle will recruit only a small number of fibers, in order to conserve energy. Have you seen that new eight-cylinder Buick, which can drive on only four cylinders when you don't need the extra power? Your muscles do pretty much the same thing.

Let me give you an idea about how muscle can affect your weight. Your body is burning calories at all times, even when you are not doing anything. This is your resting metabolic rate. Some people have a higher resting metabolic rate, which means they are burning more calories, even at rest. Some people have a lower resting metabolic rate, which means they are burning fewer calories at rest. One of the factors that determines your resting metabolic rate is the amount of muscle you have. In other words, the more muscle you have, the more calories you burn. Depending on which study you read, one pound of muscle burns anywhere from 5 to 10 calories in a 24-hour period, in its resting state, a lot more if it's active. I know this does not sound like a lot, but over time this could make a big difference in your weight.

Let's say you started strength training and gained four pounds of muscle (in addition to the muscle you gained you also stopped your body from losing muscle). This means you will burn an extra 20 to 40 calories per day, and that's in a resting state. You can lose 2 to 4 pounds of fat in a year simply by gaining four pounds of muscle, without having to do any extra activity. If you become active by doing aerobics, having more muscle means you will burn more calories during the aerobic activity.

Now, the problem with losing muscle as we age is the fact that it affects our metabolic rate, and as our metabolic rate gets slower and slower, we gain weight unless we change our eating habits. Most people notice weight gain around the age of 30, because by that time they have lost enough muscle to slow down their metabolic rate to the point where they begin gaining weight.

Since our everyday lives don't require much heavy lifting, we need to give our bodies a reason to maintain existing muscle, or to add more muscle. That is where strength training comes in. It provides the stimulus the body needs to maintain and/or build muscles. Maintaining muscle mass is essential for maintaining a higher metabolic rate, which makes weight loss easier.

Here is one more fact that you'll find very interesting, if you want to lose weight. Studies have shown that when people lose weight by dieting and aerobic training only, up to 25% of the weight they lose comes from muscle, which in turn slows down your metabolic rate and makes weight loss more difficult. Basically, trying to lose weight without doing some form of resistance training is a great way to sabotage your progress. Even if you don't gain any muscle from strength training, your metabolic rate will still increase, due to the fact that you'll stimulate your muscles to recruit more muscle fibers, which will make you stronger and, more importantly, the muscle itself will utilize more calories, which will help you lose weight.

You don't need to weight train that much in order to get benefits from your weight training routine. Lifting weights two to three times per week is ideal but even once per week is still better than nothing. One set of 10 to 15 reps for each major muscle group is fine for most beginners. Here are the major muscle groups you want to exercise: chest, upper back, shoulders, biceps (front of upper arms), triceps (back of upper arms), legs, abs, lower back. The whole weight training routine should take you no more than 20 minutes.

The importance of aerobic training

Aerobic exercise is any exercise that requires oxygen for the production of energy. The reason aerobic exercise is important to a weight loss program is that it's one of the fastest ways to burn fat, and the fastest way to improve your cardiovascular system, which is very important to overall health and well-being. Moreover, by improving your cardiovascular system, you become more aerobically fit and your body is better able to burn stored fat.

Keep in mind that even though aerobics offers great benefits, doing aerobics without doing anything else can actually sabotage your progress. For example, you can be doing plenty of aerobics and still gain weight because you're not watching your diet. Or, as I mentioned earlier, if you're trying to lose weight by doing aerobics only, up to 25% of the weight you will lose will come from muscle.

Try to stretch after each workout, to prevent your muscles from stiffening up. Hold each stretch for 15 seconds or more. The following are examples of indoor and outdoor aerobic exercises. *Outdoors:* Walking, jogging, cycling, cross-country skiing, hiking, swimming, inline skating, rowing. *Indoors:* Treadmill, stair-stepper, stationary cycle, NordicTrack, rowing machine, swimming, aerobics classes.

If you're wondering which aerobic workout burns the most calories, it doesn't really matter. All that matters is that you choose an aerobic activity you like, because the bottom line is, if you don't like a particular aerobic activity, you won't do it consistently, even if it's the "best" exercise you can do. Nor will you push yourself while you're doing it, so you won't get the maximum benefit from it anyway. So when it comes to picking aerobic activities, don't try to choose the one that burns the most calories, choose the one you enjoy the most.

I advise my clients to start with three aerobic workouts per week of 10 to 20 minutes each and work their way up to three to five aerobic workouts per week of 30 minutes each.

If you need help with developing an effective exercise routine that you can live with, I'm in the process of writing a book that covers everything you need to know about exercise and how to make exercise habitual, in the same way this book will help you make good eating habits second nature. If you would like me to notify you when the book is published, please send an e-mail to **stavros@LiveYourWayThin.com**, with "Exercise Book" in the subject line. I expect to have my exercise book published by the end of 2012.

Section 16: Healthy Recipes

I encourage you to experiment with these recipes; try different vegetables, quantities, and spices to match your taste. The vegetable quantities are all estimates. Have fun making these recipes your own!

Cannellini Bean Salad

1 lb. cannellini beans, fresh or canned (if fresh, soak in water overnight, then boil until soft)
5 scallions, chopped
3 red and/or green peppers, chopped
2 oz. olive oil (or to taste)
vinegar (to taste, optional)
pinch salt

Mix vegetables and beans, add olive oil and vinegar to taste.

Use as much or as little of each ingredient as you like, according to your taste. Don't use too much olive oil because, although a little is good for you, too much is still fattening.

This salad will stay fresh very well in the refrigerator and you can eat it cold. Make it in large amounts and have it throughout the week.

Broccoli & Red Pepper Soup

2 lbs. fresh or frozen broccoli, chopped into large pieces
2 sticks celery, coarsely chopped
1 large onion, diced
3 garlic cloves, finely chopped
3 Tbsp. dried vegetable soup mix (such as Vogue VegeBase)
1/3 cup uncooked brown rice
3 red bell peppers
juice from 1 lemon
1 Tbsp. vinegar
seasonings (to taste, but very little salt)

Step 1
In a large soup pot, combine 3 quarts of water, broccoli, celery, onion, garlic, vegetable soup mix, and rice. Simmer, covered, until broccoli is soft.

Step 2
Cut the red peppers in half and remove the seeds. Roast under a broiler or on a grill, skin side facing the heat source, until skin begins to blacken. Remove the skins and puree peppers in a blender.

Step 3
When the broccoli is soft, mash the vegetables in the pot using a potato masher. Add pureed red peppers to the pot. Add lemon, vinegar, and seasonings (e.g., tarragon, thyme, white or black pepper) to taste.

Artichoke Hearts with Peas

3 lbs. canned artichoke hearts, cut in half
4 cups frozen peas, thawed
handful fresh dill, chopped
6 scallions, chopped
1 ½ cups tomato sauce (fresh or canned)
2 Tbsp. olive oil
1 cup water (more as needed)
salt (to taste)
pepper (to taste)

Step 1
Sauté dill and scallions in olive oil for 5 minutes.

Step 2
Add the peas, and sauté for 5 more minutes.

Step 3
Add the tomato sauce, artichoke hearts, water, pepper, and very little salt. Cook until artichokes are hot.

Black-Eyed Pea Salad

For this salad, select quantities of the vegetables according to your taste.

black-eyed peas (fresh or canned; if fresh, soak in water overnight, then boil until soft)
onions, chopped
scallions, chopped
tomatoes, chopped
romaine lettuce, finely chopped
fresh dill, chopped
olive oil (to taste)
vinegar (to taste, optional)
pinch salt

Mix all vegetables with peas. Add olive oil and vinegar to taste.

Use as much or as little of each ingredient as you like. Just make sure you don't use too much olive oil because, although it is good for you, too much is still fattening.

This salad will stay fresh in the refrigerator and can be eaten cold. You can make it in large amounts and have it throughout the week.

Boiled Chicory Salad

This great side dish is easy to make and is very good for you. It can be eaten hot or cold, so you can make it ahead of time and keep it in the refrigerator.

1 bunch chicory
olive oil (to taste)
lemon juice (to taste)
pinch salt

Step 1
Cut the root off the chicory and wash the chicory.

Step 2
Boil in slightly salted water until the stem is soft (about 30 minutes).

Step 3
Strain chicory, cut into bite-sized pieces.

Step 4
Add olive oil, lemon juice, salt. Mix and serve.

Mediterranean-Style Lima Beans

1 lb. bag dry lima beans (soak in water overnight)
2 cups tomato sauce
2 Tbsp. olive oil
1 medium onion, chopped
2 cloves garlic, chopped
3 Tbsp. fresh parsley, chopped
oregano (to taste)
pinch salt
pepper (to taste)

Step 1
Boil beans with a little salt, until they are soft, but not too soft (about 45 minutes).

Step 2
Heat oven to 350 degrees. Put olive oil in a skillet and sauté the onions, garlic, and oregano 3 to 4 minutes. Add the parsley, salt, pepper, and tomato sauce, and continue cooking another 10 minutes.

Step 3
Once beans are done, drain them, *reserving some of the cooking liquid*.

Step 4
Put the beans in an ovenproof pan and add the tomato mixture.

Step 5
Add reserved water from the boiled beans, until beans are nearly covered. Mix and put in the oven for about 40 minutes.

Peas & Corn

1 onion, chopped
2 cloves garlic, chopped
3 cups mushrooms, any variety, diced
1 can peeled whole tomatoes in juice, chopped
2 cups frozen peas, thawed
1 cup frozen corn, thawed
oregano (to taste)
1 Tbsp. olive oil
black pepper (to taste)
pinch salt
bay leaves (1 if whole, a pinch if chopped)

Step 1
Put olive oil in large pan and sauté the onions and garlic for 3 minutes.

Step 2
Add mushrooms and sauté for 3 minutes.

Step 3
Add chopped tomatoes with the juice. Add oregano, black pepper, salt, and bay leaves. Bring to a boil.

Step 4
Once boiling, add peas and corn and cook 10 to 15 minutes, uncovered, until peas and corn are cooked.

Ratatouille

1 eggplant, cubed
2 zucchini, cubed
2 green and/or red peppers, diced large
1 large onion, diced
1 medium-sized can whole tomatoes, coarsely chopped
2 Tbsp. olive oil
1 clove garlic, chopped
oregano (to taste)
pepper (to taste)
pinch salt

Step 1
Sauté onions with the olive oil, garlic, salt, pepper, and oregano, until onions are translucent.

Step 2
Add the tomatoes and cook 5 minutes.

Step 3
Add the eggplant and cook for about 10 minutes.

Step 4
Add the zucchini and peppers and cook until the vegetables are done.

Red Beet Salad

This easy-to-make side dish is very good for you. It can be eaten hot or cold, so you can make it ahead of time and keep it in the refrigerator.

1 bunch fresh beets with their greens
olive oil (to taste)
vinegar (to taste)
pinch salt

Step 1
Peel the beets and cut them in halves or quarters, depending on how big they are.

Step 2
Wash beet greens, put them in a pot with the beets, and fill with water.

Step 3
Boil until beets are fork-tender (about 30 minutes). Strain and put beets and greens in a bowl.

Step 4
Add little olive oil, vinegar to taste, a little salt, and mix.

Spinach & Rice

4 lbs. spinach, stems removed
handful fresh dill, chopped
9 scallions, chopped
4 Tbsp. olive oil
7 cups tomato juice
2 cups chicken stock
1 14-oz. box instant brown rice
oregano (to taste)
pinch salt
pepper (to taste)

Step 1
In a large pot, sauté the scallions and dill in the olive oil.

Step 2
Add the oregano, salt, pepper, brown rice. Sauté 1 minute.

Step 3
Add the tomato juice and chicken stock, bring to a boil, and stir in the spinach. Reduce heat and simmer covered, stirring occasionally to prevent sticking (*Note:* if you are using thawed frozen spinach, wait until the rice is almost cooked before adding it.) Cook until the rice is done.

Spinach with Onions

1 lb. spinach
1 large onion, thinly sliced
2 cloves garlic, finely chopped
1 Tbsp. olive oil
oregano (to taste)
pepper (to taste)
pinch salt

Step 1
In a pot, sauté the onions and garlic in the olive oil until onions are translucent.

Step 2
Add the spinach and the spices, and cook until spinach is done.

Greek-Style Tomato Salad

2 ripe tomatoes, cut in wedges
1 green pepper, thinly sliced
½ red onion, thinly sliced
oregano (to taste)
salt (to taste)
3 Tbsp. olive oil (or to taste)
2 slices feta cheese (optional)

Mix ingredients in a bowl and serve. If possible, allow the salad to sit for 30 minutes to allow the flavors to mingle.

Eggplant & Beans (main course)

1 eggplant, peeled and diced
1 onion, thinly sliced
1 green pepper, diced
1 Tbsp. lemon juice
3 Tbsp. ketchup
very little olive oil
2 cups garbanzo or other beans, cooked or canned
½ onion, finely chopped (optional)

Step 1
Steam the eggplant for 10-12 minutes. (If you don't have a steamer, put eggplant in a pot with a little water and cover. Make sure you stir it often so it won't stick.)

Step 2
Wet a napkin with a little olive oil and wipe the cooking surface of a pan with it. Sauté the sliced onion and pepper over low heat in a covered skillet for 6-8 minutes.

Step 3
Add the steamed eggplant, lemon juice, and ketchup and simmer, uncovered, another 5 minutes. Add the beans, cook until hot, and add the chopped onion right before you take the skillet off the heat.

Mushroom & Onion Mix (side dish)

3 cups mushrooms, any variety, diced
1 onion, diced
1 to 2 Tbsp. dried vegetable soup mix such as Vogue VegeBase (to taste)

Wet a napkin with a little olive oil and wipe the cooking surface of a pan with it. Sauté the onions and mushrooms 5 minutes and add the vegetable soup mix. Cook until done.

Eggplant Patties (main course or side dish)

2 eggplants, peeled and sliced
3 Tbsp. balsamic vinegar
4 cloves garlic, finely chopped
1 cup fat-free, low sodium vegetable stock
1 Tbsp. rosemary, finely chopped
pinch black pepper
pinch oregano
1 Tbsp. Bragg's Liquid Aminos

Step 1
Heat oven to 350 degrees. Slice eggplant into 1/3 inch thick patties.

Step 2
Mix the remaining ingredients in a flat-bottomed bowl.

Step 3
Wet a napkin with a little olive oil and wipe down a nonstick baking tray or sheet of aluminum foil, creating a thin coating of oil.

Step 4
Dip the eggplant patties in the spice mixture for 5 seconds, then place on the oiled tray or foil.

Step 5
Bake eggplant for 20-25 minutes. Mushrooms can be used instead of, or in addition to, the eggplant.

Dip for Eggplant Patties (optional)

½ cup mayonnaise (you can substitute fat-free or 50% reduced fat mayonnaise)
Garlic, finely chopped (to taste)

Mix the mayonnaise and garlic.

Tip: Do not dip the vegetables directly into the dip because you'll end up with too much. Instead, dip the tip of your bare fork in the dip, and eat your vegetables with it. This way, you'll get the taste of the dip, without overpowering the vegetables or consuming too much fat.

Vegetable Scrambled Eggs

2 eggs (free range or organic)
8 oz. Rancho Fiesta Style Vegetables, thawed
1 cup feta cheese, cut in small cubes
½ cup onions, chopped
½ cup tomatoes, chopped
1 Tbsp. olive oil
salt (to taste)
pepper (to taste)

Step 1
Heat olive oil in a pan and add the chopped onions. Cook 4 minutes.

Step 2
Add the chopped tomatoes. Cook 2 minutes.

Step 3
Add the thawed vegetables and cook until hot. (Cover the pan to heat the vegetables faster.)

Step 4
Beat the eggs in a bowl, mix in the feta cheese, and add mixture to pan. Season with salt and pepper. Keep mixing until eggs are fully cooked.

Note: To reduce the fat, remove one of the egg yolks before you beat the eggs.

Spinach Salad with Tuna

4 ½ oz. fresh baby spinach
1 cup water-packed canned tuna
1 cup diced cucumber
½ cup canned corn
¼ cup chopped scallions
1 Tbsp. olive oil
1 Tbsp. balsamic vinegar

Mix ingredients in a large bowl and serve.

Village-Style Black-Eyed Pea Salad

2 cups canned black-eyed peas, rinsed and well drained (if using fresh beans,
soak in water overnight, then boil until soft)
2 cups diced red pepper
1 cup diced cucumber
½ cup chopped scallions
¼ cup chopped dill
2 Tbsp. olive oil
2 Tbsp. vinegar
salt (to taste)

Mix ingredients in a large bowl and serve.

Romaine Lettuce Salad with Dill

1 head romaine lettuce
1 cup chopped scallions
½ cup chopped fresh dill
2 Tbsp. olive oil
2 to 3 Tbsp. vinegar (to taste)
salt (to taste)

Step 1
Cut romaine lettuce thinly, on the diagonal.

Step 2
Mix ingredients in a large bowl and serve.

Section 17: Conclusion and Final Thoughts

There are no secrets to losing weight and getting in shape. There is no magic pill that will help you lose weight, nor will there ever be one. The truth is, weight loss will take some effort on your part. Only permanent changes in your daily habits will result in permanent weight loss. In order to lose weight and get into shape, all you need to do is implement a balanced resistance training routine (two to three times per week), an aerobic training routine (four to five times per week), and the 7 Eating Habits I introduced in this book. You have to be consistent in your efforts if you want to get results.

Any weight loss program that does not include strength training, aerobic training, and proper nutrition is doomed to fail. A program that promises weight loss with little or no effort on your part is deceiving you. If it were that easy to lose weight, everybody would be thin by now. Keep in mind that weight loss is not everything. Being healthy is far more important. Losing weight in an unhealthy way will only harm you in the long run.

Confucius said it best, and for that reason I would like to repeat his quote: "A journey of a thousand miles begins with a single step." A journey of a thousand miles can seem overwhelming, but when you focus on one single step at a time, it becomes a much easier proposition. Your journey toward achieving a lean and healthy body begins with changing a single habit.

Let me tell you a story that perfectly demonstrates how focusing on one small step can make a big difference in your life. As you might already know, many people have a hard time flossing regularly. Despite the fact that flossing is very beneficial and doesn't take more than five minutes, most people don't seem to be able to stick to the task regularly. For years, I was one of these people. I would go to my dentist for a cleaning and he'd lecture me on the importance of flossing and all the bad things that could happen to my teeth if I didn't floss regularly. I'd leave the dentist's office determined to start flossing every night from then on.

But once I got home, I'd floss regularly for few weeks and then, for whatever reason, I'd stop. At my next checkup, it would be the same routine. The dentist would tell me that if I didn't floss enough, bad things would happen to my teeth, I'd get motivated for few weeks, but then I would stop flossing again. This went on for years.

One day I thought to myself, how am I supposed to motivate people to develop good exercise and eating habits, when I can't even get myself to stick to the habit of flossing daily? The answer came to me when I came across the kaizen method, which helps people implement change in their lives through small, easy steps.

Kaizen is a Japanese word that means, "change for the better." The kaizen method was first used in Japan after World War II, by companies like Toyota, in an attempt to improve all functions of the company by taking small but continuous steps. We all know how well Japanese industry — especially the automobile industry — did after World War II. The kaizen method played a big part in that rapid turnaround. I decided I would try the kaizen way to get myself flossing regularly.

I started flossing one tooth every night. I must admit, I did feel a little silly flossing only one tooth, but I stuck to my task. Night after night, I flossed one tooth. Every person I told about my strange new habit told me that I wasn't getting any benefit from flossing only one tooth. My response was that I was not trying to floss, I was trying to *develop the habit* of flossing, and by keeping the action so small, it was almost impossible not to do it. Every so often, when I felt like it, I'd add one more tooth to floss. One day I realized I was flossing every tooth! It's been over six years since then, and flossing has become an automatic action that I do every night without a second thought.

If you want to lose weight and keep it off permanently, good eating habits also have to become automatic. The only way to make good eating habits automatic is to introduce them into your life one at a time, just like I did with flossing one tooth at a time. Once you've made good eating habits automatic, you'll never have to worry about your weight again, thanks to your new way of healthful eating.

If you have any questions or comments about my program, please don't hesitate to e-mail me at stavros@liveyourwaythin.com. I look forward to hearing your success story!

For Further Reference and Reading

American Council on Exercise. *Personal Trainer Manual.* San Diego, CA: American Council on Exercise, 1996.

Ballentine, Rudolph. *Diet and Nutrition: A Holistic Approach.* Honesdale, PA: The Himalayan Institute Press, 1978.

Beck, Judith S. *The Beck Diet Solution*, 2007. Birmingham, AL: Oxmoor House, 2007.

Cordain, Loren. *The Paleo Diet.* New York: John Wiley and Sons, 2002.

Diamond, Harvey. *The Fit for Life Solution.* St Paul, MN: Dragon Door Publications, 2002.

Diamond, Harvey and Marilyn. *Fit For Life.* New York: Warner Books, 1985.

Diano, Sabrina, et al. *Ghrelin controls hippocampal spine synapse density and memory performance.* New York, NY: Nature Neuroscience, 2006.

Faigin, Rob. *Natural Hormone Enhancement.* Cedar Mountain, NC: Extique Publishing, 2000.

Fuhrman, Joel. *Eat To Live.* New York: Little, Brown and Company, 2003.

Hofmekler, Ori. *The Warrior Diet.* St Paul, MN: Dragon Door Publications, 2001.

Maltz, Maxwell. *The New Psycho-Cybernetics.* New York: Prentice-Hall, 2001.

Maurer, Robert. *One Small Step Can Change Your Life: The Kaizen Way.* New York: Workman, 2004.

Roizen, Michael. and La Puma, John. *The Real Age Diet.* New York: HarperCollins, 2001.

Shelton, Herbert M. *The Hygienic System: Orthotrophy.* Dr. Shelton's Health School, 1975

Tilden, J.H. *Toxemia Explained.* Pomeroy, WA: Health Research Books, 1960.

Acknowledgments

First, I would like to thank the most important people in my life: My wife Svetlana, my son Alexander, and my daughter Arina, for their understanding and support while I was writing this book. I worked many long days trying to finish it, which took away a lot of our time together.

Another person to whom I owe everything to is my mother, Iris Mastrogiannis, who supported me through all the ups and downs of my life and my career. I would also like to thank the rest of my family, the Rountos and Beretis, because without their support my personal training business might not even exist.

Many people have helped in the creation of my weight loss program and in the writing of *Eat It All By Eating Right*. I would especially like to thank my clients at Olympus Personal Training & Weight Management, because without their input and the trust they put in me, this book would never have been written. The other person I would like to thank is Becky Schoenfeld for the great job she did editing this book and for going beyond what I expected from her. She was a great influence on the look and feel of this book.

The following people, although I have never met them in person, have had a great impact on my life. Their inspiration, through their books and tapes, has kept my motivation alive throughout the seemingly endless research that went into developing and writing *Eat It All By Eating Right*. Thank you, Anthony Robbins, Doran J. Andry, and Joseph McClendon III.

About the Author
Stavros Mastrogiannis
Founder & Personal Trainer, Olympus Personal Training & Weight Management

Stavros Mastrogiannis, founder of Olympus Personal Training & Weight Management Center in Danbury, Connecticut, is a 19-year veteran in the weight loss field, empowering clients with a unique, life-changing perspective. Stavros resided in Greece for 12 years before moving to the United States in 1987. After moving to the U.S., Stavros continued to visit Greece where, over time, he observed changes in Greek eating habits, exercise habits, and daily living, resulting in a national weight problem similar to that which exists in the U.S.

At age 21, Stavros made the decision to shift gears, from the pursuit of a career in preparing fine cuisine, to the weight loss and fitness profession, where felt he could make a difference in peoples' lives. He is committed to putting an end to widespread weight loss misinformation, and to helping people lose weight the healthy way.

Stavros founded Olympus Personal Training & Weight Management Center in 1996. His approach to fitness stresses the importance of developing a realistic regimen of exercise and nutrition that can be maintained for a lifetime of good health. His exceptional understanding of motivation and consistency as the root of success in long-term fitness has enabled him to teach hundreds of people how to effectively lose weight and keep it off, even when other trainers and diet plans have failed.

Stavros provides his clients with cutting-edge nutrition and weight loss information from the top medical institutes. He is a source of inspiration for thousands, having organized the Danbury Weight Loss Challenge in 2004 and having partnered with St. Jude Children's Hospital in Memphis, TN for the Get In Shape for 2007 Challenge.

Prior to founding Olympus Personal Training & Weight Management Center, Stavros was a fitness instructor for the

Regional YMCA of Western Connecticut and Newtown Health & Fitness Club. In these positions, Stavros enjoyed educating, training, and motivating his clients as they pursued their weight loss and fitness goals.

Stavros holds an A.O.S. in Culinary Arts from the Culinary Institute of America. He received a diploma in Fitness and Nutrition from International Correspondence Schools and holds numerous certifications, including CPR, Nutrition Specialist, and ACE (American Council on Exercise) certifications as a Personal Trainer and Lifestyle & Weight Management Consultant.

45239091R00066